Psychiatric Pharmacosciences of Children and Adolescents

The
PROGRESS IN PSYCHIATRY
Series

David Spiegel, M.D.,
Series Editor

Psychiatric Pharmacosciences of Children and Adolescents

Edited by
Charles Popper, M.D.

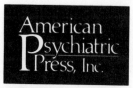

American
Psychiatric
Press, Inc.

1400 K Street, N.W.
Washington, DC 20005

Copyright © 1987 American Psychiatric Press, Inc.
ALL RIGHTS RESERVED
Manufactured in the United States of America
First Edition

The paper used in this publication meets the minimum requirements of American National Standard for Information Sciences—Permanence of Paper for Printed Library Materials, ANSI Z39.48-1984.   ∞

Library of Congress Cataloging-in-Publication Data

Psychiatric pharmacosciences of children and adolescents.

(The Progress in psychiatry series)
Includes bibliographies.
1. Pediatric psychopharmacology. I. Popper, Charles,
1946–   . II. Series. [DNLM: 1. Brain—drug effects.
2. Brain—growth & development. 3. Psychopharmacology—
in adolescence. 4. Psychopharmacology—in infancy &
childhood. QV 77 P965]
RJ504.7.P77   1987   615'.78'088054   86-28826
ISBN 0-88048-089-0 (alk. paper)

Contents

Contributors

Ross J. Baldessarini, M.D.
Interim Director, Laboratories for Psychiatric Research, Mailman Research Center, McLean Hospital; and Professor of Psychiatry and in Neuroscience, Harvard Medical School

Joseph T. Coyle, M.D.
Distinguished Service Professor of Child Psychiatry; Director, Division of Child Psychiatry; and Professor of Psychiatry, Neuroscience, Pharmacology, and Pediatrics, The Johns Hopkins Medical Institutions

Joel Herskowitz, M.D.
Assistant Professor of Pediatrics and Neurology, Boston University School of Medicine

Peter I. Jatlow, M.D.
Chief of Laboratory Medicine, Yale-New Haven Hospital; Chairman and Professor, Department of Laboratory Medicine; and Professor of Psychiatry, Yale University School of Medicine

Silvio J. Onesti, M.D.
Director, Hall-Mercer Children's Center, McLean Hospital

Charles Popper, M.D.
Director, Child and Adolescent Psychopharmacology, Hall-Mercer Children's Center, McLean Hospital; and Clinical Instructor in Psychiatry, Harvard Medical School

Martin H. Teicher, M.D., Ph.D.
Group Leader, Developmental Psychopharmacology Program, Mailman Research Center; Director of Outpatient Psychopharmacology, Adult Outpatient Clinic, McLean Hospital; and Assistant Professor of Psychiatry, Harvard Medical School

Introduction to the
Progress in Psychiatry Series

The *Progress in Psychiatry* Series is designed to capture in print the excitement that comes from assembling a diverse group of experts from various locations to examine in detail the newest information about a developing aspect of psychiatry. This series emerged as a collaboration between the American Psychiatric Association's Scientific Program Committee and the American Psychiatric Press, Inc. Great interest was generated by a number of the symposia presented each year at the APA Annual Meeting, and we realize that much of the information presented there, carefully assembled by people who are deeply immersed in a given area, would unfortunately not appear together in print. The symposia sessions at the Annual Meetings provide an unusual opportunity for experts who otherwise might not meet on the same platform to share their diverse viewpoints for a period of three hours. Some new themes are repeatedly reinforced and gain credence, while in other instances disagreements emerge, enabling the audience and now the reader to reach informed decisions about new directions in the field. The *Progress in Psychiatry* Series allows us to publish and capture some of the best of the symposia and thus provide an in-depth treatment of specific areas which might not otherwise be presented in broader review formats.

Psychiatry is by nature an interface discipline, combining the study of mind and brain, of individual and social environments, of the humane and the scientific. Therefore, progress in the field is rarely linear—it often comes from unexpected sources. Further, new developments emerge from an array of viewpoints that do not necessarily provide immediate agreement but rather expert examination of the issues. We intend to present innovative ideas and data that will enable you, the reader, to participate in this process.

We believe the *Progress in Psychiatry* Series will provide you with an opportunity to review timely new information in specific fields of interest as they are developing. We hope you find that the excitement of the presentations is captured in the written word and that this book proves to be informative and enjoyable reading.

David Spiegel, M.D.
Series Editor
Progress in Psychiatry Series

Foreword

In searching for the causes of medical disorders, we have long known to encompass and synthesize knowledge of the biological, psychological, behavioral, and social components of the structure and function of the mind and body. Human structure and function is ever changing, vastly in the fetus, greatly in the child and adolescent. As we observe the continuous and reciprocal interactions of individual with environment, we are following developmental transformations of structures and functions.

This book on the science of developmental psychopharmacology is a contribution to basic pharmacology and the biology of human behavior. The authors take psychiatry a step further toward the goal of achieving a scientific developmental psychopathology and a related system of therapy. Popper and his colleagues set forth important aspects of what is known about development of the brain in its relationship to the pharmacological treatment of thought, emotion, and action. Psychiatrists will be better able to identify the subcellular as well as the interpersonal mechanisms that are involved in the development and appearance of psychiatric disorder.

Biological studies in pediatric psychiatry have led to advances for the benefit of adults and children. Drug treatments of attention deficit–hyperactivity disorder are now being used to treat its residual form in late adolescence and adulthood. Clonidine treatment of Tourette's disorder was originally developed by child psychiatrists, and is now in widespread usage in adult psychiatry. The development of new treatments in all of psychiatry is strengthened as the field of child and adolescent psychopharmacology moves ahead.

Baldessarini has noted a resistance to experimentation in child psychiatry as a major factor hampering the growth and refinement of new treatments. Psychiatrists' attitudes toward protecting the development of the child have been complemented by a new sense of protection: Research and innovation are seen as essential and beneficial to the children and adolescents themselves.

Psychiatrists will welcome this timely and instructive book as an excellent and lasting resource. As the basic and clinical sciences in adolescent and child psychiatry contribute new insights into developmental features of mental disorders and their treatments, people of all ages will benefit.

Silvio J. Onesti, M.D.

Introduction

This is the first book that brings together, for the practicing psychiatrist, the array of pharmacological sciences that underlie child and adolescent psychopharmacology. This is not a "how-to" book for managing clinical treatments, but a clinician's log of the developmental underpinnings of neuroscience and pharmacology.

After many years of waiting for the gains of the biological psychiatry movement, children now are benefiting from fast-moving changes in clinical psychopharmacology. In the psychiatric treatment of adolescents and children, there is a broadening use of medications. New indications for "old" or traditional psychotropic medications are being defined in children. Over the last 10 years, there has been rapid expansion in the clinical use of antidepressants and lithium in children and adolescents. In many parts of the country, "empirical trials" have proceeded at a time when only scanty data are available in the medical literature to advise and guide treatment.

Underlying the rapid advancement in clinical pediatric psychopharmacology, there have been major gains in basic developmental neurobiology and developmental pharmacology. Several areas of pharmacological and developmental science will be reviewed in this volume: the biochemical development of the brain, developmental pharmacokinetics, developmental pharmacodynamics, and long-term effects of drugs on the development of the body and brain. In the face of many medical unknowns in these fields, the ethics of using psychopharmacological treatments for children will be considered from a clinical point of view.

In the first chapter, Dr. Coyle describes the biochemical development of the brain, emphasizing the development of neurotransmitter systems in the brain stem. Although other components are surely critical in brain development, concepts of neurotransmitter development contribute to current theorizing about psychiatric disorders.

At present, only a small fraction of neurotransmitters have been studied, and only a small portion of brain has been mapped. We have more information about rat brain than human brain. Yet some general neurodevelopmental principles may be identified. One basic principle is the responsiveness of the developing biochemical structure of the brain to environmental influences and experiences.

At the level of hypothesis, it appears that at least certain neurotransmitters have a "trophic" influence on the development of other neurotransmitter systems and on the biochemical organization of the brain. There may be some "fetal neurotransmitters" whose use during development is more prominent than later, and whose function may be related to activities of fetal life.

In the future, more direct studies of human brain may be possible. At present, we have only a small number of clinical studies, which permit us to confirm hypotheses generated in biochemical studies of laboratory animals.

In the human fetus, brain development begins early in gestation, and great complexity is uncovered even in the simplest studies. By the end of the first trimester, the major neurotransmitter systems may be identified by the presence of biogenic amines in simple nuclei that are the origins of developing neuronal systems (Masudi and Gilmore 1983; Nobin and Bjorklund 1973). Brain development proceeds at different paces in different neurotransmitter systems in different parts of the human neocortex (Figure 1).

The biochemical development of the human brain continues beyond childhood, at least into late adolescence, and merges into the slowly evolving neurochemical changes of adult life. There is no clear completion date or end point of neurochemical development.

The age-related changes in the pharmacokinetic handling of drugs describe a different "developmental line" of immediate clinical relevance. The major message of Dr. Jatlow's chapter on developmental aspects of drug disposition is that children typically need higher doses of medications than expected on the basis of adult psychopharmacology. After correction for body weight, upward adjustments of 50 to 100 percent relative to adult doses are commonly needed to overcome the rapid drug biotransformation evident into mid- or late adolescence.

Pediatricians could have told psychiatrists many years ago that higher doses of antidepressants would be needed to treat depressed children, but this piece of pharmacological knowledge was not applied in psychiatric practice or research until the late 1970s. His-

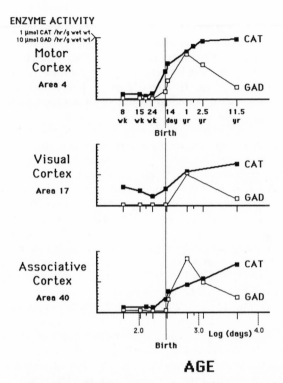

Figure 1. Developmental changes of neurotransmitter-synthesizing enzymes in different regions of human neocortex (based on data presented by Diebler et al. [1979]).

Acetylcholine- and GABA-synthesizing enzymes show different patterns of change in three regions of the cerebral cortex during human development. Enzymatic activity was sampled at autopsy at various ages from early fetal life to 11.5 years. Human brain regions include motor, visual, and associative (gyrus supramarginalis) cortex. Choline acetyltransferase (CAT) is the rate-limiting enzyme in the synthesis of acetylcholine, and glutamate decarboxylase (GAD) is involved in GABA synthesis.

CAT activity is high in the visual cortex during early fetal life and declines by end of the second trimester. In other areas, there is low CAT activity during the first 6 months of gestation. By birth, CAT activity shows a generalized and substantial increase, which continues through the prepubertal years and into adulthood.

GAD activity is low in the fetus, but increases specifically in the motor cortex by the day of birth. There are peak levels of GAD activity in all three cortical areas at age 1 year and a subsequent decline during childhood.

Patterns of biochemical change during development depend on brain region, neurotransmitter system, and age.

torically, psychiatrists gave "conservative" doses of medications to children, resulting in the undertreatment of a generation of depressed children and contributing to the delayed recognition of the usefulness of antidepressants for treating affective disorders in children. We now know to use age-corrected doses of liver-metabolized drugs in the routine pharmacological treatment of adolescents and children.

Developmental pharmacokinetics has more to offer clinical practice: the value and limits of therapeutic drug monitoring, corrections for "atypical" metabolizers, dosage adjustments around puberty, managing effects of varying exercise and diet on drug levels in blood, and dose optimization. This knowledge is technical, but is not complicated and is of direct value to clinicians.

After "correcting" for developmental pharmacokinetic effects, it is possible to identify certain effects of psychotropic agents as age-dependent. These age-related drug-induced phenomena can be clues to the shifting chemical or physiological organization of the body or brain. The chapter of Drs. Teicher and Baldessarini summarizes the current state of knowledge of developmental pharmacodynamics in humans and in laboratory animals.

In humans, clinical examples of developmental pharmacodynamic effects include age-related effects of amphetamine on arousal and behavioral activity, extrapyramidal motor reactions of neuroleptics, and possibly mood changes induced by steroids. In animals, experimental studies on a broader range of pharmacological agents are possible. By combining pharmacological, biochemical, and behavioral studies in laboratory animals, it has been possible to define the sequential activation of various neurotransmitter systems during development. The age-related activation of different neurotransmitter systems may be crucial to understanding the appearance of normal behaviors and the pathogenesis of certain psychiatric disorders of children and adults. A neurochemical-developmental theory of behaviors and diseases permits a conceptual approach to developing new treatment strategies.

A major clinical concern regarding the use of medications in adolescents and children is the potential risk of long-term damage to the body and the development of the brain. Dr. Herskowitz's review of developmental toxicology and neurotoxicology surveys the broad range of drugs used in medicine, neurology, and psychiatry. The largest class of these drug-induced "developmental" effects may be prevented by ordinary medical attentiveness to side effects during management.

There are five main examples of age-related biological effects of drugs on development: psychostimulants (slowing of body growth), aspirin (Reye's syndrome), tetracycline (organ discoloration), and probably hexachlorophene (impairment of myelin formation) and valproate (hepatotoxicity).

These examples range from mild to severe, but perhaps the most striking feature is their small number compared to the large array of drugs used throughout medicine. Contrary to usual clinical expectation, it appears that children's growing bodies and brains are not very much more sensitive than adults to toxic effects of drugs—except for the uniquely vulnerable period of intrauterine development.

Of these five drugs, two (valproate and psychostimulants) were used at first predominantly in children. Because of this, a prior record in adults of adverse reactions, special properties, and effects on a wide variety of biological mechanisms was unavailable. It is strongly advised that, where possible, psychiatrists employ medications in children only after there is significant experience of their use in adults.

Because antidepressants, neuroleptics, and lithium have been used in adults for more than two decades, careful introduction of these agents for treatment of children may now be considered acceptable (or even overdue). We may infer that the risks of unpredicted major developmental toxicity will probably be quite low. Nonetheless, during the introduction of these medications to the child and adolescent population, careful observations of possible toxicological effects—guided by our prior knowledge of their effects in adults—will be needed.

The final chapter on ethics may seem to be an unusual choice for inclusion in this volume on pharmacosciences, but it appears here because of its "basic" position in our clinical thinking: Underlying current pharmacological treatments of children, there are many unknowns regarding biochemical development, pharmacokinetics and pharmacodynamics, and possible long-term toxicological effects. These unknowns influence physicians' treatment recommendations and highlight ethical and legal problems in clinical decision making.

This final chapter elaborates a clinician's thinking on the justification of clinical psychopharmacological treatments of children and adolescents when the biological risks of these treatments are partially undetermined. Since the *relative* risks of the drug treatments and the psychiatric diseases are undefined, we would be ill-advised to assume that the drugs are necessarily more toxic than the psychiatric diseases they are employed to treat. The Food and Drug Administration guidelines, designed for regulating the advertising of pharmaceutical manufacturers, do not attempt to limit or direct physicians' judgments about the clinical use of drugs in children. We are left to our professional judgments to make thoughtful decisions for the benefit of the individuals we treat. There is the additional challenge of effectively involving parents and children in complicated medical decisions, where clinically crucial data on both drugs and diseases are lacking.

These problems are not answered by delaying drug treatment or waiting for a child to grow past a biochemically vulnerable stage: biochemical development and somatic vulnerability are lifelong. Withholding a drug because of medical unknowns becomes a disservice to patients when we have probabilistic knowledge about the risks of the future course of the psychiatric disease. There is no "safe way" around these ethical issues in child and adolescent psychopharmacology: there are only sensible judgments to be made in dealing with these dilemmas.

The interaction of social and environmental factors with the biological and somatic is a repeated theme throughout this volume. It might be considered a "basic" premise that the need for pharmacological therapy in a child or adolescent typically implies the need for psychosocial interventions aimed at other developmental gains. Since disruption in one dimension of development frequently leads to "multiaxial" problems, even these pharmacological essays contribute support to the notion of a multimodal approach to the correction of developmental problems and the need for multidimensional thinking in facilitating the attainment of personal goals.

Charles Popper, M.D.

REFERENCES

Diebler MF, Farkas-Bargeton E, Wehrle R: Developmental changes of enzymes associated with energy metabolism and the synthesis of some neurotransmitters in discrete areas of human neocortex. J Neurochem 32:429–435, 1979

Masudi NA, Gilmore DP: Biogenic amine levels in the mid-term human fetus. Dev Brain Res 1:9–12, 1983

Nobin A, Bjorklund A: Topography of the monoamine neuron systems in the human brain as revealed in fetuses. Acta Physiol Scand (Suppl 388) 88:1–40, 1973

Chapter 1

Biochemical Development of the Brain: Neurotransmitters and Child Psychiatry

Joseph T. Coyle, M.D.

Chapter 1

Biochemical Development of the Brain: Neurotransmitters and Child Psychiatry

Psychodynamic, social, and cognitive theories have stressed the importance of developmental stages in normal maturation and the failure to master these stages in the genesis of psychiatric disorders. From a biomedical perspective, biological ontogenetic events and the impact of brain insults during maturation are viewed as contributing to the vulnerability to and the appearance of neuropsychiatric disorders. More recently, there is increasing evidence of critical interactions of neurobiological factors with psychological and environmental events in the etiology of psychiatric disorders.

Chemical neurotransmitters appear to function as the mediators of the effects of virtually all psychotropic medications (Cooper et al. 1986; Coyle 1985). Because the biochemical processes involved in synaptic neurotransmission play a critical role in normal as well as pathological brain function, it stands to reason that understanding neurochemical ontogeny is an essential part of psychiatry.

The ontogeny of these biochemical processes is intimately tied to emergence of behaviors, developmental stages, and the age-related appearance of psychiatric disorders such as attention deficit-hyperactivity disorder, affective disorders, Tourette's disorder, autistic disorder, and schizophrenia.

Current knowledge of the development of neurotransmitter systems in the brain will be reviewed, with an emphasis on the neurons of the reticular core, which are located in the brain stem. There are other dimensions of the biochemical development of the brain, in-

Joseph T. Coyle, M.D., receives support from the Surdna Foundation and an NIMH Research Career Development Award (MH-00125). The excellent secretarial assistance of Alice Trawinski is gratefully acknowledged.

cluding structural and vascular elements, that may pertain to neuropsychiatric abnormalities. However, this chapter attempts to relate information regarding the development of neurotransmitter systems to understanding the onset of psychiatric disorders.

SYNAPTIC NEUROTRANSMISSION

Although discussed elsewhere in detail (Coyle 1985), the concepts involved in synaptic neurotransmission will be briefly reviewed. The transferral of information from the receptive area of neurons, the dendritic extensions of their cell bodies, down the axon to the synaptic terminals occurs by a means of electrical-chemical wave of depolarization (Figure 1). However, the communication between neurons

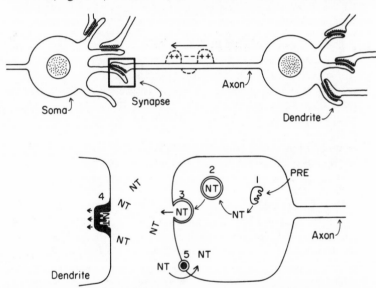

Figure 1. Schematic representation of synaptic transmission. *Top:* The structural components of the neuron include the soma (cell body), the receptive extensions known as dendrites, the axon, and the specialized contact between the axon terminal and dendrite known as the synapse. *Bottom:* The processes involved in chemical synaptic transmission at the synapse are illustrated. Precursors (PRE) for the neurotransmitter (NT) are taken up into the terminal and converted by enzymes to the neurotransmitter (1). The neurotransmitter is stored in vesicles (2) for release (3) into the synaptic cleft, where it interacts with receptors (4) on the dendrite. In many cases, the neurotransmitter is inactivated by reuptake (5) into the nerve terminal.

at their synaptic contacts occurs by chemical messengers, known as neurotransmitters, that are released by the nerve terminals when a wave of depolarization reaches them. Neurotransmitters can be divided into different classes based on their mode of synthesis and their neurophysiological effects.

With regard to mode of synthesis, neuropeptides represent one rapidly expanding class of neurotransmitters, whose synthesis is directed by processes within the neuronal cell body dependent on messenger ribonucleic acid (mRNA). The precursor neuropeptide, translated from the mRNA, is modified by a series of enzymatic reactions to yield the active neuropeptide. The active neuropeptide is then accumulated within vesicles and transported down the axon to the nerve terminal, where the active neuropeptide is released on depolarization. A second class, the "simple" or nonpeptide neurotransmitters, includes biogenic amines, amino acids, and certain other substances. Their synthesis is regulated by enzymes contained within the nerve terminal. In this latter case, neurotransmitter synthesis is not closely tied to translational events at the neuronal cell body but is controlled at the level of the nerve terminal, and therefore is much better able to respond to rapid changes in neurotransmitter demand. Nevertheless, synthetic enzymes themselves are dependent on mRNA-regulated processes within the neuronal cell body.

The neurotransmitter released by a given neuron is used throughout all its axonal extensions and terminal ramifications, in essence conferring on the neuron a biochemical identity. The neuron contains the biochemical processes necessary to synthesize, store, release, and inactivate the neurotransmitter. Conversely, the neuron does not usually possess the biochemical processes required for the synthesis of other neurotransmitters. An important exception to this rule is the growing evidence of co-localization of neurotransmitters: there now is a rapidly increasing number of systems consisting of neurons that contain two neurotransmitters. Generally, this involves a combination of a neuropeptide and a nonpeptide transmitter such as a biogenic amine. Neurons that use specific neurotransmitters tend to be grouped together in clumps of cell bodies known as "nuclei" or to have laminar-specific distributions in cortical structures.

The neurotransmitter receptors mediate postsynaptic responses. The neurotransmitter receptors translate the message encoded in the neurotransmitter in a highly specific interaction similar to the relationship between a key (the neurotransmitter) and a lock (receptor-transducer). These effects can be divided into three broad categories: excitatory, inhibitory, and modulatory. This simple tripartite division does not adequately address the complex and variable relationships between the neurotransmitter receptors, on the one hand, and various ion channels and enzymatic processes that mediate the neuronal effects of the neurotransmitters, on the other. Excitatory or inhibitory response represents the "hard" information communicated in the brain (e.g., the decision as to whether a receptive neuron fires). Neuromodulators such as the biogenic amines and several neuropeptides appear to alter neuronal responsiveness to excitatory or inhibitory inputs.

The rapidly increasing number of substances in the brain thought to serve as neurotransmitters is now approaching 50 (Table 1). However, neurotransmitters that at present have been implicated in the pathophysiology of psychiatric disorders or in the mechanism of action of psychotropic medications are much more restricted in number. This fact undoubtedly reflects our current state of ignorance; nevertheless, for the sake of clarity, the following discussion will focus on the small group of neurotransmitters so far involved in explaining disease processes or drug effects.

THE RETICULAR CORE

A particularly important class of neurons implicated in the mechanisms of action of several classes of psychotropic drugs have their cell bodies located in the reticular core. The reticular core neurons are distributed in the midbrain and brain stem, and have highly diffuse and arborized axonal projections that innervate large areas of the nervous system, particularly the forebrain. The location of the cell bodies in the reticular core ensures that they receive diverse input from neuronal systems coming from the periphery and from neuronal systems projecting down from the forebrain to lower brain regions. This anatomical organization emphasizes the integrative role of the reticular core, which broadly regulates the activity of neurons in the cerebral cortex, striatum, and limbic system. Consistent with this anatomic organization, neurophysiological studies suggest that the reticular core neuronal systems "modulate" neuronal activity in the cortex and related structures rather than conveying precise bits of excitatory or inhibitory information to discrete neurons within these regions.

Noradrenergic Neurons

The primary source of noradrenergic innervation of the cerebral cortex, limbic system, midbrain, and cerebellum is the locus coeruleus, a small group of pigmented neurons situated bilaterally on the floor of the fourth ventricle under the cerebellum (Figure 2). These neurons use norepinephrine as their neurotransmitter, which is syn-

Table 1. Partial List of Putative Neurotransmitters in the Brain

Acetylcholine	**Neuropeptides (continued)**
Monoamines	*Pituitary opiomelanocortins*
dopamine	alpha-melanocyte-
norepinephrine	stimulating
epinephrine	hormone (α-MSH)
serotonin	β-MSH
histamine	γ-MSH
phenylethanolamine	corticotropin (ACTH)
octopamine	β-lipotropin (β-LPH)
Amino Acids	γ-LPH
γ-aminobutyric acid (GABA)	α-endorphin
γ-hydroxybutyrate	β-endorphin
glutamate	γ-endorphin
glycine	dynorphin
taurine	leu-enkephalin
asparate	met-enkephalin
Neuropeptides	*Other peptides*
	substance P
Hypothalamic hormones	angiotensin II
vasopressin	neurotensin
oxytocin	bombesin
somatostatin	vasoactive intestinal
arginine-vasotocin	peptide (VIP)
thyrotropin-releasing	delta sleep-inducing
hormone (TRH)	peptide (DSIP)
luteinizing-hormone-	gastrin-cholecystokinin
releasing hormone	series
(LHRH)	glucagon
	carnosine
	bradykinin
	Other Substances
	growth homone
	prolactin
	adenosine
	prostaglandins
	corticosteroids
	estrogens
	androgens
	catecholestrogens

thesized from the amino acid tyrosine within the nerve terminals. The postsynaptic effects of norepinephrine are mediated by alpha receptors and beta receptors. Whereas beta receptors are coupled to adenylate cyclase and use cyclic adenosine monophosphate (cAMP) as their intracellular effector, alpha receptors may be linked to membrane ion channels. The noradrenergic neuronal cell bodies send axons that innervate virtually all neurons in the cerebral cortex and limbic system; accordingly, an individual noradrenergic neuron may contact up to 10^8 other neurons. The noradrenergic neuronal systems have been implicated in arousal, anxiety, and mood.

Serotonergic Neurons

Located somewhat more anterior to the locus coeruleus in the midbrain are the cell bodies of the serotonergic neurons situated in the raphe nuclei (Figure 3). These neurons use the indoleamine serotonin as their neurotransmitter, which is synthesized from the essential amino acid tryptophan by enzymes contained in the nerve terminal.

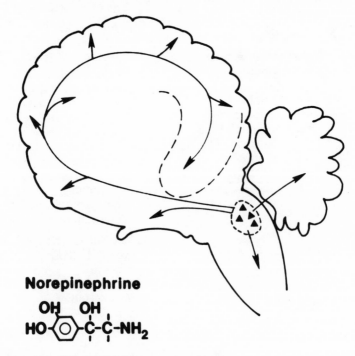

Norepinephrine

$$HO-\bigcirc-\overset{\overset{\displaystyle OH}{|}}{C}-\overset{\overset{\displaystyle OH}{|}}{C}-NH_2$$

Figure 2. Noradrenergic neuronal pathways.

Interestingly, the circulating levels of tryptophan are below the concentration that saturates the biosynthetic enzyme for serotonin, so fluctuations in serum tryptophan levels directly affect brain serotonin content (Wurtman 1983). Similar to the noradrenergic neurons, the serotonergic neurons provide an extremely diffuse innervation to the striatum, entire cortex, and limbic system. Recent evidence indicates that the dual input by noradrenergic and serotonergic neurons may interact in modulating neuronal activity (Stockmeier et al. 1985). The serotonergic neurons have been implicated in mood, aggression, and rapid eye movement (REM) sleep.

Dopaminergic Neurons

Situated more anteriorally in the base of the midbrain is a group of pigmented neurons located in the substantia nigra that utilize dopamine as their neurotransmitter (Figure 4). Dopamine is synthesized by enzymes contained within their nerve terminals from the amino acid tyrosine. The dopamine neurons in the substantia nigra proper

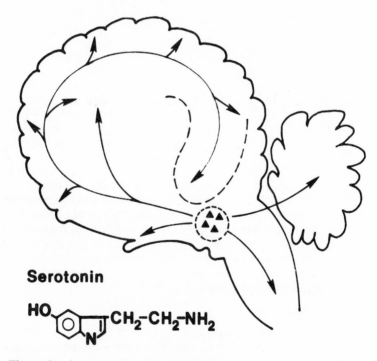

Serotonin

$$HO-\bigcirc\!\!-\!\!\bigcirc_N\!\!-\!CH_2\!-\!CH_2\!-\!NH_2$$

Figure 3. Serotonergic neuronal pathways.

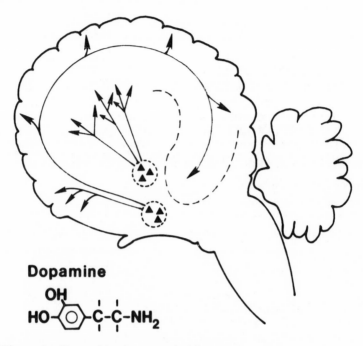

Figure 4. Dopaminergic neuronal pathways.

provide a very diffuse and massive innervation to the corpus striatum, which consists of the caudate and putamen. It is estimated that 15 percent of the nerve terminal synapses in the striatum are dopaminergic. This system plays a critical role in modulating motor activity as evidenced by the symptoms of Parkinson's disease, which results from a selective degeneration of the dopaminergic neurons. A more medially located group of dopamine neurons innervates the limbic system and the frontal cortex. Notably, this pathway has the neuropeptide cholecystokinin co-localized within it, whereas the lateral nigrostriatal dopamine projection does not contain this neuropeptide. There is indirect evidence supporting the notion that the mesocortical-limbic dopamine neurons play a role in reward systems, attention, and cognitive integration.

Cholinergic Neurons

The most anterior component of the reticular core consists of the cholinergic neurons, whose cell bodies are scattered from the base of the midbrain overlying the hypothalamus anterior to the medial

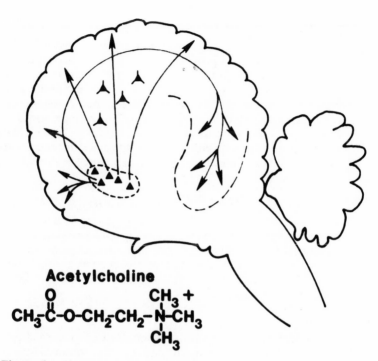

Acetylcholine

$$CH_3-\overset{\overset{\displaystyle O}{\|}}{C}-O-CH_2-CH_2-\overset{\overset{\displaystyle CH_3}{|}}{\underset{\underset{\displaystyle CH_3}{|}}{N}}{}^+-CH_3$$

Figure 5. Cholinergic neuronal pathways.

septum (Figure 5). The cholinergic neurons release acetylcholine as their neurotransmitter, which is synthesized within the nerve terminals from choline. These neurons provide a diffuse innervation to all areas of the cerebral cortex, hippocampus, and limbic system. Studies of Alzheimer's disease show a striking degeneration of cholinergic (as well as norepinephrine and somatostatin) neurons, indicating that this cholinergic pathway plays an important role in memory and perhaps in other higher cognitive functions (Coyle et al. 1983).

GABAergic Neurons

Within the cerebral cortex, local circuit neurons that have their cell bodies and synaptic connections restricted to the cortex play a critical role in processing information. These neurons, because of their location, are not components of the reticular core. A major class of these neurons utilizes γ-aminobutyric acid (GABA) as their neurotransmitter, which is synthesized from the amino acid L-glutamic acid. GABA is the primary inhibitory neurotransmitter in the brain, and may be released by up to 30 percent of brain synapses. The GABAergic neurons intrinsic to the cortex are scattered throughout all cortical layers, and provide important inhibitory input into the pyramidal cells, the primary output system from the cortex. The GABA receptors mediating the effects of this neurotransmitter are linked to receptor sites for the benzodiazepines. A number of anti-convulsants interact directly with the GABA receptor, and anxiolytic benzodiazepines indirectly enhance the sensitivity of the GABA receptor to its neurotransmitter. Pharmacological evidence indicates that GABAergic neurons are involved in seizure susceptibility, sedation, and anxiety.

GENERAL PRINCIPLES OF BRAIN DEVELOPMENT

Brain development can be likened to a symphony with the emergence of an overall theme punctuated by brief percussive events that provide the critical driving rhythm (Jacobson 1978). Brain development at the cellular level can be divided into four primary events: neuroblast (cell) division, neuronal migration, transmitter-specific differentiation, and synaptogenesis (Figure 6).

Cell Origin

The source of immature neurons are nests of epidermal germinal cells that typically lie within the center of the primordial brain. The

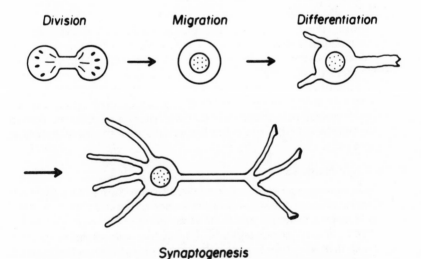

Synaptogenesis

Figure 6. Critical events in neuronal development in brain.

dividing neuroblasts generate immature postmitotic neurons that make up the nervous system. Neuroblast cell division is not a continuous process; it involves discrete regions and synchronized periods of cell multiplication. There is a precisely timed and localized sequence in the pattern of formation of the brain, with the most primitive and caudal being laid down first, and more recently evolved structures (e.g., the cerebral cortex) appearing in subsequent "bottom-to-top" steps.

Neuronal Migration

The postmitotic immature neuron typically migrates from the germinal zone, through intermediate sites, to its final resting place within the brain. In the brain stem, discrete populations of neurons grouped together in "nuclei" are generated during a brief period of mitotic activity, migrate together, and coalesce into functionally circumscribed neuronal cell groupings. The noradrenergic locus coeruleus, the dopaminergic substantia nigra, and the serotonergic raphe nuclei are examples of biochemically specific homogenous nuclei within the brain stem. In cortical structures that have a laminar organization, the early formed immature neurons migrate to the surface, and the subsequently formed neurons are layered on top of them. Thus cortical development occurs by an "inside-to-outside" sequence.

The guideposts that direct the migration of these immature neurons remain to be characterized. Certain types of glial cells may serve as scaffolding; trophic factors released from target sites may point the direction; and neuron-neuron interactions in transit appear to provide local cues.

Neurotransmitter Choice

The appearance of the specialized biochemical mechanisms responsible for neurotransmitter synthesis generally takes place after the immature neuron has reached its final destination. In most neuronal systems studied in detail, there is a coordinate and concurrent expression of these biochemical processes, including the biosynthetic enzymes, storage/release processes, and transport mechanisms for the neurotransmitters. The immature neuron appears to be fully capable of releasing its neurotransmitter well before it has elaborated axons and developed mature synaptic contacts. This finding has led to the speculation that neurotransmitters may serve as trophic factors or "hormonal" cues in the very immature nervous system.

Recent studies have provided evidence that immature neurons, in a chameleon-like fashion, may transiently manifest the biochemical characteristics typical for one neurotransmitter before assuming the neurotransmitter characteristics that they will retain throughout their mature life (Katz et al. 1983). For example, certain immature migrating neurons in the gut transiently manifest an enzyme that synthesizes catecholamines, tyrosine hydroxylase, and a catecholamine uptake process before they differentiate into peptidergic neurons.

This transient expression of transmitter metabolic machinery reflects the pluripotential of the immature neurons that has been elegantly described in studies of the sympathetic neuroblasts (Patterson 1978). When the immature sympathetic ganglion is grown in tissue cultures with an organ that receives predominantly parasympathetic (cholinergic) innervation, a trophic factor is released into the medium that causes the neurons to manifest cholinergic characteristics. If nerve growth factor, a trophic peptide resembling pro-insulin, is added to the medium, the neurons assume noradrenergic characteristics. Finally, addition of corticosteroids to the culture medium stimulates the synthesis of the enzyme that converts norepinephrine to epinephrine as in the adrenal medulla.

The factors that control the phenotypic expression of neurotransmitter characteristics in brain neurons remain poorly understood at present. However, recent studies indicate that nerve growth factor stimulates the development of forebrain cholinergic neurons (Mobley et al. 1985).

Synaptogenesis

The final process of brain development involves the elaboration of the primary receptive portion of the neuron (the dendrites) and the communicational portion of the neuron (the axon), leading ultimately to the formation of synaptic contacts. The length of axonal projections may be limited to a few millimeters or less, as is the case for local circuit GABAergic neurons in cortex, or up to a meter, as is the case for noradrenergic and serotonergic projections descending from the midbrain to innervate the spinal cord.

Although the bulk of synaptogenesis occurs during the early stages of brain development (e.g., before 2 years of age in humans), it is becoming increasingly apparent that the elaboration and modification of axonal-dendritic synaptic contacts continue to a much more limited degree throughout adulthood. In fact, a critical feature of senescence may be the loss of ability to develop new synaptic contacts.

Numerous experiments have revealed a remarkable neuroanatomical precision in the formation of axonal contacts. Studies in the frog indicate that transsection of the optic nerve and rotation of the eye, after a critical period of development, will result in regrowth of axons to reinnervate the appropriate target neurons in the geniculate with remarkable fidelity (Jacobson 1978). In the rodent, an hereditary disruption of the normal laminar distribution of neurons within the cerebral cortex does not prevent the ultimate development of appropriate synaptic connections between the thalamus and the maldistributed cortical pyramidal cells (Caviness and Rakic 1978). Nevertheless, serotonergic and noradrenergic components of the reticular core appear to be relatively insensitive to the integrity of their postsynaptic neurons within the cerebral cortex, and will develop a quantitatively normal terminal arbor in the absence of a full complement of cortical neurons (Johnston et al. 1979).

In summary, evidence obtained thus far in fundamental developmental neurobiological studies indicates that the maturation of the nervous system is a remarkably complicated process that involves an interplay between precisely timed developmental events that are orchestrated by genetically determined programs. Because of the limited information contained in the cellular deoxyribonucleic acid (DNA), all developmental events cannot be seen as directly controlled by the genes but rather are also determined by cell-cell interactions. There is growing evidence that neurotransmitters themselves may be intimately involved in the intercellular communication that regulates the development of neuronal systems. Genetic defects or environmental insults that occur in the period of neurogenesis, during the first trimester in humans, are associated with gross teratogenic or structural defects in brain development. Later-appearing genetically expressed disturbances or environmental insults are more likely to affect the emerging neuronal connectivity in the brain.

DEVELOPMENT OF BRAIN NEUROTRANSMITTERS

The most detailed studies on development of specific neurotransmitter systems in brain have been carried out in the laboratory rat. The reticular core neurons (e.g., the noradrenergic, dopaminergic, serotonergic, and cholinergic neuronal systems) are located in the brain stem and are among the neuronal systems that are formed early in development. In contrast, the GABAergic interneurons within the cortex are formed later in brain development during the genesis of the cerebral cortex. For these neuronal systems, the limited information currently available from studies in the developing human and subhuman primate brain suggest that the general principles defined in the rat may be applicable to the human.

Norepinephrine

The noradrenergic neurons of the locus coeruleus are among the most caudal components of the reticular core and are formed particularly early in brain development. The locus coeruleus issues from a brief period of intense cell division, which lasts approximately 36 hours in the rodent (Lauder and Bloom 1974). This nucleus is established in the rodent brain when the brain represents less than 1 percent of the adult weight, which is equivalent to the middle of the first trimester of pregnancy in humans (i.e., approximately 6 weeks gestational age). As this nucleus coalesces, all the intraneuronal structures and biochemical processes required for the synthesis, storage, and release of norepinephrine appear simultaneously—in a coordinate rather than a sequential fashion. The nascent axons that grow from the newly formed noradrenergic neurons contain norepinephrine; noradrenergic axons are among the very earliest to appear in the primordial cerebral cortex during its formation. Although noradrenergic terminals contribute a very small percentage of the total number of synaptic contacts in the adult cerebral cortex, up to 30 percent of the synapses in the immature cortex may be noradrenergic at this early stage of development (Coyle and Molliver 1977).

This early and transient developmental predominance of noradrenergic terminals in cortex raises the possibility that the pioneering noradrenergic innervation may play a critical role in the formation and differentiation of the cerebral cortex. Indeed, lesions of the noradrenergic system early in development affect synaptic plasticity in the cortex, the process whereby cortical synaptic contacts are altered on the basis of sensory input. For example, chemical depletion of catecholamines prevents the developmental shift in ocular dominance after monocular occlusion in young kittens (Kasamatsu and Pettigrew 1976).

The noradrenergic input to the primordial cortex is subsequently diluted by the development of other cortical inputs such as the thalamocortical pathways as well as the elaboration of the rich synaptic arbors of neurons intrinsic to cortex.

It is important to make a distinction between the relative contribution of noradrenergic input at early developmental stages and the total elaboration of noradrenergic processes throughout the brain with maturation. Although the noradrenergic input to the cortex is relatively large early in the development, the volume of the cortex is quite small at this time. With the progressive increase in cortical volume with maturation, the noradrenergic terminal arbor expands accordingly. Thus the small group of noradrenergic neuronal cell bodies in the locus coeruleus elaborates a remarkably arborized group of axons and terminals, which then develop in conjunction with the brain regions that they innervate.

Serotonin

The serotonergic neurons located in the raphe nuclei in the midbrain, anterior to the locus coeruleus, are formed somewhat later in brain development than the noradrenergic system. Like the noradrenergic neurons, the serotonergic neurons send axons to virtually all areas of the fetal nervous system. The early innervation of the primordial cortex by serotonergic neurons also appears to modulate cortical development because the pharmacological disruption of the serotonergic neuronal system alters the rate of cell division in the fetal cerebral cortex (Lauder and Krebs 1976). In contrast to the noradrenergic system, the serotonergic innervation of the cerebral cortex develops much more gradually despite its early appearance in the cortex (Lidov and Molliver 1982).

Dopamine

The dopaminergic neurons, located in the substantia nigra even more anterior in the midbrain, are formed during a brief period of cell division in the late first trimester in humans, and then send axons to the primordial striatum. Although the striatal innervation by the dopaminergic afferents is particularly dense in adulthood, accounting for 15 percent of the striatal synapses, and is virtually confluent when viewed by histofluorescent techniques that reveal the neurotransmitter itself, the initial input to the striatum consists of islands of dopaminergic innervation (Graybiel et al. 1981). These islands of dopaminergic innervation appear to be organizational foci for striatal development because their presence corresponds to areas of ingrowth of other striatal inputs and of cell division activity of striatal intrinsic neurons. These initial outposts of striatal dopaminergic innervation gradually expand with maturation to achieve the confluent pattern observed in the adult striatum.

Quantitative neurochemical studies indicate that striatal dopaminergic innervation develops quite slowly and reaches its apex around puberty in rats as well as in humans.

The development of the more medially located dopaminergic neurons, whose axons innervate the limbic system as well as the frontal and cingulate cortex, is not well understood. This system, however, also exhibits a gradual development that continues on past late childhood into adolescence.

Acetylcholine

The most anterior components of the reticular core are the cholinergic neurons of the basal forebrain complex. Reflected by the large size and anterior-posterior expanse of these nuclei, the neurons of the cholinergic complex undergo division over a prolonged period of time, continuing later in development than the more caudal components of the reticular core. Nevertheless, the cell bodies in cholinergic basal forebrain complex are formed well in advance of the development of their target areas of innervation in the cortex, hippocampus, and limbic system. In contrast to the early appearance of noradrenergic and serotonergic fibers in the primordial cortex, invasion by cholinergic axons is delayed. In the rodent, cholinergic innervation does not occur until a full week after birth, and the limited information from studies with primate cortex suggests that the development of cholinergic innervation to cortex peaks during the first year of life (Coyle and Yamamura 1976). As the cortical cholinergic projections appear to be the last developing components of the reticular core, there is a basis for speculation that this input may play a role in finalizing or cementing synaptogenesis in the cortex.

γ-Aminobutyric acid

In contrast to the neuronal components of the reticular core, the cortical GABAergic neurons are local circuit neurons. The neuroblast progenitors for the cortical GABAergic neurons reside in the subcortical periventricular germinal zone, and generate immature GABAergic neurons throughout the period of cortical formation, consistent with the fact that the GABAergic neurons are located in virtually all cortical layers. The appearance of GABAergic neurons occurs much later in brain development than the reticular core neurons. The period of GABAergic neuronal maturation coincides with the progressive differentiation of neurons within the cerebral cortex.

Synaptic neurochemical studies, however, indicate that the biochemical components involved in the synthesis, release, and inactivation of GABA do not develop in a coordinate fashion seen in the noradrenergic, serotonergic, and dopaminergic systems (Coyle and Enna 1976). The levels of GABA in the immature brain are disproportionately high, in contrast to the relatively low activity of its synthetic enzyme glutamic acid decarboxylase. At early stages of development, the high affinity uptake-inactivation process for GABA surpasses the activity in adulthood. In contrast, the postsynaptic GABA receptors and their modulatory benzodiazepine receptors exhibit a much more gradual developmental increase in the cerebral cortex. The physiological implications of the developmental disparities in the pre- and postsynaptic components of the GABAergic system remain unclear at present.

DEVELOPING NEUROTRANSMITTER SYSTEMS AND HUMAN PSYCHOPATHOLOGY

Conclusive evidence of the involvement of specific neurotransmitter systems in any major psychiatric disorder has yet to be established. The integration of our current knowledge on the development of brain neurotransmitter systems into concepts about the pathophysiology of major mental disorders must remain highly speculative. Nevertheless, because of the clear role played by neurotransmitters in the mechanism of action of psychotropic drugs effective in the treatment of several neuropsychiatric disorders, there is adequate justification for some preliminary speculation.

Norepinephrine

It seems appropriate that the noradrenergic neuronal system, which appears to mediate arousal and anxiety, two primitive defenses necessary for survival, would appear at the earliest stages of brain development. Indeed, the noradrenergic system is represented in the brains of the lowest vertebrates on the phylogenetic tree.

In the first year of infant development, arousal, fear of strangers, and separation anxiety emerge early in the behavioral repertoire. Pharmacological studies in immature rat and monkey provide evidence that central noradrenergic systems are critically involved in separation-distress behaviors (Harris and Newman 1987). The role of cortical noradrenergic input in modulating synaptic plasticity and modifiability early in development provides a basis for speculation about the relationship between affect-laden experiences in infancy and their effects on the establishment of the synaptic organization of the cortex.

The noradrenergic system has also been implicated in the pathophysiology of mood disorders and the action of antidepressant drugs. The last decade has witnessed mounting evidence of the occurrence of major depressive disorder in adolescents and in prepubertal children (Kovacs et al. 1984). These juvenile depressive episodes can have cognitive and physiological features similar to those in adults, including anhedonia, suicidal preoccupation, and abnormal dexamethasone suppression tests (Puig-Antich and Weston 1983). Furthermore, these mood disorders in children respond to antidepressant treatment in a manner similar to that in adults. The vulnerability to severe mood disturbances, as evidenced by marasmus and anaclitic depression, may occur even in infancy. The early development of the noradrenergic system provides a neuronal basis for theorizing about these clinical findings.

Serotonin

The serotonergic system, in addition to its potential role in mood disorders, has long been implicated in the pathophysiology of infantile autism. Consistent with the establishment of serotonergic innervation of cortical and limbic structures during fetal life, the symptoms of autistic disorder (infantile autism) appear within the first 18 months of life.

Over the last decade, there have been several reports of elevated levels of serotonin in whole blood in a significant portion of individuals suffering from autistic disorder (Young et al. 1982). Geller et al. (1983) reported that fenfluramine, a drug that enhances central serotonergic neurotransmission, caused both behavioral and cognitive improvement in several children with autistic disorder. The general clinical efficacy of this pharmacological strategy to alter central serotonergic neurotransmission in autistic disorder, however, remains unresolved (August et al. 1984). Todd and Ciaranello (1985) demonstrated the presence of auto-antibodies both in serum and in the cerebrospinal fluid against one subtype of brain serotonin receptor. Approximately 40 percent of the autistic individuals tested exhibit this receptor antibody, whereas the incidence is quite low in controls.

Thus infantile autism, a complex disorder or group of disorders, may be the developmental consequence of early serotonergic dysfunction.

Dopamine

The dopaminergic system has long been implicated in the pathophysiology of attention deficit-hyperactivity disorder. Stimulants that enhance central dopaminergic neurotransmission, such as d-amphetamine and methylphenidate, reduce motor activity and increase attention span in these children. Neuroleptics that block dopamine receptors can also reduce the hyperactivity, although their effects on cognitive functions may be less salutory (Werry and Aman 1975). Shaywitz and colleagues (1976) demonstrated that neonatal destruction of the dopaminergic neurons results in a marked enhancement of the normally increased motoric activity of prepubescent rat pups, and that this hyperactivity can be reduced by administration of stimulants.

The gradual development of striatal-limbic dopaminergic pathways may account for the age-related emergence of symptoms of Tourette's disorder and schizophrenia. Tourette's disorder, whose symptoms include hyperactivity, motor tics, and vocal tics, typically emerges between ages 5 and 12 years. The symptoms of the disorder are exacerbated by stimulants that enhance dopaminergic neurotransmission and are attenuated by neuroleptics that block dopamine receptors; therefore, the emergence of symptoms may result from the altered development of dopaminergic neurotransmission. In light of evidence of decreased levels of the dopamine metabolite homovanillic acid in the cerebrospinal fluid of Tourette patients, there is reason to believe that the syndrome involves an increased postsynaptic response to dopamine, possibly due to a supersensitivity of the dopamine receptors (Singer et al. 1982).

Schizophrenia with onset in childhood represents merely an earlier appearance of the disorder, which typically has its onset in mid to late adolescence, according to studies using the diagnostic criteria of DSM-III (American Psychiatric Association 1980). These criteria include the characteristic "positive" symptoms, such as hallucinations, delusions, and thought disorder, which are most responsive to antidopaminergic neuroleptic medications (Crow 1980). The clinical antipsychotic potencies of different neuroleptic agents are tightly correlated with their in vitro blockade of D_2 dopamine receptors (Creese et al. 1976, Seeman et al. 1976). Positron emission tomography (PET) reveals elevated D_2 dopamine receptor density in the caudate nuclei of nonmedicated schizophrenics in vivo (Wong et al. 1986). The neuroleptic-responsive (D_2 dopamine receptor-correlated) positive symptoms of schizophrenia may appear on an age-related continuum, beginning in childhood but peaking in late adolescence when dopamine levels in the forebrain have reached their apex (Kendler et al. 1982).

Acetylcholine

Clinical psychopharmacological studies in humans and lesion studies in experimental animals have implicated the forebrain cholinergic projections in higher cognitive functions, especially memory (Coyle et al. 1983). In humans, the postnatal development of cholinergic innervation to the cerebral cortex and hippocampal formation occurs concurrently with the emergence of complex cognitive functions such as speech and memory in the infant at the end of the first year of life. The demonstration of selective impairments in cortical and hippocampal cholinergic integrity in Alzheimer's dementia has highlighted the role of this cholinergic system in cognitive disorders.

Evidence of rather selective cortical cholinergic deficits has been found in middle-aged individuals with Down's syndrome who exhibit the neuropathology of Alzheimer's disease (Price et al. 1982). A genetic connection between Down's syndrome and Alzheimer's disease has recently been demonstrated using recombinant DNA techniques, which have revealed a marker on chromosome 21 in some individuals with Alzheimer's disease (St. George-Hyslop et al. 1987). While the structural integrity of these cholinergic pathways in younger Down's individuals, who do not exhibit the pathology of Alzheimer's disease, remains to be determined, there is pharmacological evidence of a compromised cholinergic system in young people with Down's syndrome (Coyle et al. 1986). Studies on the fetal brain of a certain mouse mutant, characterized by trisomy of the genes encoded on chromosome 21 in humans, indicate an impaired development of the cholinergic neurons (Singer et al. 1984).

Dysfunction of selective aspects of cortical cholinergic projections might conceivably contribute to mental retardation of some children and to the selective cognitive deficits of some children with hereditary and acquired learning disorders.

Peptide Neurotransmitters in the Brain

Since the original description of peptide transmitters in the 1970s, a rapid pace of research in brain peptides has been simultaneously pursued in both basic pharmacological and clinical studies. At present, the neuronal localization of most of these peptides in the brain is poorly understood, and the development of pre- and postsynaptic elements of the peptidergic neurons remains inadequately characterized in humans and in animals. Nevertheless, preliminary findings suggest a role for neuropeptides in regulating brain development. For example, under certain experimental conditions in the newborn rat, the proliferation of axonal branches of monoamine neurons in brain may be modified by excitatory substance P neurons and by inhibitory enkephalin neurons (Jonsson and Hallman 1982). Thus brain peptides may be able to exert "trophic" influences on the monoamine systems during development, and speculatively may be involved in explanations of certain psychiatric and neurological disorders.

Dysfunction of endogenous opiate peptide systems has been hypothesized in a number of psychiatric disorders, including affective illness, anxiety disorders, and anorexia nervosa. Given the lengthy list of other neuropeptides that are thought to serve as neurotransmitters (Table 1, p. 7), it may be anticipated that future research will uncover a considerable array of neuropsychiatric disorders associated with chemical pathology of the peptide neurotransmitter systems in the brain.

CONCLUSION

Over the last decade, considerable advances have been made in our understanding of the neuroanatomical and neurochemical processes of brain development. These advances have occurred in the context of a rapid expansion in the identification and characterization of the substances involved in chemical synaptic neurotransmission. While information is regrettably scanty regarding the development of neurotransmitter systems in the human (and subhuman primate) brain, neuroanatomical studies suggest some general validity for extrapolation from observations in the rodent.

Current findings point to intriguing relationships beween the development of components of the reticular core neuronal systems and the emergence of age-related behavioral and psychiatric disorders. These relationships provide heuristically valuable leads that may assist us in our better understanding of the pathophysiology of psychiatric disorders.

In addition, these findings suggest ways in which early developmental experiences may affect cortical maturation, and provide an experimental context to integrate the biopsychosocial approach to psychiatry. The emerging understanding of brain neurotransmitter ontogeny may lead to the development of more rational treatments of developmentally based psychiatric disorders.

REFERENCES

American Psychiatric Association: Diagnostic and Statistical Manual of Mental Disorders, 3rd ed. (DSM-III). Washington, DC, American Psychiatric Association, 1980

August GJ, Raz N, Papanicolau N, et al: Fenfluramine treatment in infantile autism. J Nerv Ment Dis 172:604–611, 1984

Caviness VS, Rakic P: Mechanisms of cortical development: a view from mutations in mice. Annu Rev Neurosci 1:297–326, 1978

Cooper J, Bloom FE, Roth R: The Biochemical Basis of Neuropharmacology. New York, Oxford Press, 1986

Coyle JT: Introduction to the world of neurotransmitters and neuroreceptors, in Psychiatry Update: American Psychiatric Association Annual Review, Vol 4. Edited by Hales RF, Frances AJ. Washington, DC, American Psychiatric Press, 1985

Coyle JT, Enna SJ: Neurochemical aspects of the ontogenesis of GABAergic neurons in the rat brain. Brain Res 111:119–133, 1976

Coyle JT, Molliver ME: Major innervation of newborn rat cortex by monoaminergic neurons. Science 196:444–447, 1977

Coyle JT, Yamamura H: Neurochemical aspects of the ontogensis of cholinergic neurons in the rat brain. Brain Res 118:429–440, 1976

Coyle JT, Oster-Granite ML, Gearhart JD: Neurobiologic consequences of Down's syndrome. Brain Res Bull 16:773–787, 1986

Coyle JT, Price D, DeLong MR: Alzheimer's disease: a disorder of cortical cholinergic innervation. Science 219:1184–1190, 1983

Creese I, Burt DR, Snyder SH: Dopamine receptor binding predicts clinical and pharmacological potencies of antischizophrenic drugs. Science 192:481–483, 1976

Crow TJ: Positive and negative schizophrenia symptoms and the role of dopamine. Br J Psychiatry 137:383–386, 1980

Geller E, Ritvo ER, Freeman BJ, et al: Preliminary observations on the effect of fenfluramine on blood serotonin and symptoms in three autistic boys. N Engl J Med 307:165–168, 1983

Graybiel AM, Pickel VM, Joh TH, et al: Direct demonstration of a correspondence between dopamine islands and acetylcholinesterase patches in the developing striatum. Proc Natl Acad Sci USA 78:5871–5875, 1981

Harris JC, Newman JD: Alpha-2 adrenergic receptor involvement in squirrel monkey vocal behavior, in Animal Models of Anxiety. Edited by Newman JD. New York, Raven Press, 1987 (in press)

Jacobson M: Developmental Neurobiology. New York, Plenum Press, 1978

Johnston MV, Grzanna R, Coyle JT: Abnormally dense noradrenergic innervation of rat neocortex follows fetal treatment with methyazoxymethanol. Science 203:435–469, 1979

Jonsson G, Hallman H: Modulation of 6-hydroxydopamine induced alteration of the postnatal development of central noradrenaline neurons. Brain Res Bull 9:635, 1982

Kasamatsu T, Pettigrew JD: Depletion of brain catecholamines: failure of ocular dominance shift after monoculary occlusion in kittens. Science 194:206–209, 1976

Katz DM, Markey KA, Goldstein M, et al: Expression of catecholaminergic characteristics by primary sensory neurons in the normal adult rat in vivo. Proc Natl Acad Sci USA 80:3526–3530, 1983

Kendler KS, Gruenberg AM, Strauss JS: An independent analysis of the Copenhagen sample of the Danish adoption study of schizophrenia. Arch Gen Psychiatry 39:1257–1261, 1982

Kovacs M, Feinberg TL, Crouse MA, et al: Depressive disorders in childhood: a longitudinal study of the risk for a subsequent major depression. Arch Gen Psychiatry 41:643–649, 1984

Lauder JM, Bloom FE: Ontogeny of monoamine neurons in the locus coeruleus, raphe nuclei and substantia nigra of the rat. J Comp Neurol 155:469–482, 1974

Lauder JM, Krebs H: Effects of p-chlorophenylalanine on time of neuronal origin during embryogenesis in the rat. Brain Res 107:638–644, 1976

Lidov H, Molliver ME: An immunocytochemical study of the development of serotonergic neurons in the rat CNS. Brain Res Bull 8:389–430, 1982

Mobley WC, Rutkowski JL, Tenekoon GI, et al: Choline acetyltransferase activity in striatum of neonatal rats increased by nerve growth factor. Science 229:284–287, 1985

Patterson PH: Environmental determination of autonomic neurotransmitter functions. Annu Rev Neurosci 1:1–17, 1978

Price DL, Whitehouse PJ, Struble RG, et al: Alzheimer's disease and Down's syndrome. Ann NY Acad Sci 396:145–164, 1982

Puig-Antich J, Weston B: The diagnosis and treatment of major depressive disorder in childhood. Annu Rev Med 34:231–245, 1983

Seeman P, Lee T, Chau-Wong M, et al: Antipsychotic drug doses and neuroleptic/dopamine receptors. Nature 261:717–719, 1976

Shaywitz BA, Klopper JH, Yager RD, et al: Paradoxical response to amphetamine in developing rats treated with 6-hydroxydopamine. Nature 261:153–155, 1976

Singer HS, Butler IJ, Tune LE, et al: Dopamine dysfunction in Tourette syndrome. Ann Neurol 12:361–366, 1982

Singer HS, Tiemeyer M. Hedreen JC, et al: Morphologic and neurochemical studies of embryonic brain development in murine Trisomy 16. Dev Brain Res 15:155–166, 1984

St. George-Hyslop PH, Tanzi RE, Polinsky RJ, et al: The genetic defect causing familial Alzheimer's disease maps on chromosome 21. Science 235:885–890, 1987

Stockmeier CA, Martino AM, Kellar KJ: A strong influence of serotonin axons on β-adrenergic receptors in rat brain. Science 121:323–326, 1985

Todd RD, Ciaranello RD: Demonstration of inter- and intraspecies differences in serotonin binding sites by antibodies from an autistic child. Proc Natl Acad Sci USA 82:612–616, 1985

Werry JS, Aman MG: Methylphenidate and haloperidol in children: effects on attention, memory and activity. Arch Gen Psychiatry 32:790–796, 1975

Wong DF, Wagner HN, Tune LE, et al.: Positron emission tomography reveals elevated D_2 dopamine receptors in drug-naive schizophrenics. Science 234:1558–1563, 1986

Wurtman RJ: Behavioral effects of nutrients. Lancet 1:1145–1148, 1983

Young JG, Kavanaugh ME, Anderson GM, et al: Clinical neurochemistry of autism and associated disorders. J Autism Dev Disord 12:147–156, 1982

Chapter 2

Psychotropic Drug Disposition During Development

Peter I. Jatlow, M.D.

Chapter 2

Psychotropic Drug Disposition During Development

Considerable medical attention has been focused on drug disposition at the extremes of the human life cycle: in the newborn and the elderly. It is well established that the pharmacokinetics of many drugs differ from the "normal" in these age groups, and most physicians are aware that dosing regimens should be modified accordingly.

There is a significant medical literature describing the pharmacokinetic characteristics of newborns and the premature. Newborns demonstrate reduced clearance for many drugs when compared to older infants, children, and adults. However, in childhood between the period of late infancy and adolescence, there are relatively few hard kinetic data that quantify drug absorption, distribution, and elimination.

The limited developmental information on drug disposition that is available, both anecdotal and documented in the literature, is consistent: In comparison to adults, children and adolescents require larger, not smaller, weight-adjusted doses of many drugs to achieve comparable blood levels and therapeutic effects (Briant 1978; Gibaldi 1984; Morselli 1977; Morselli and Pippenger 1982; Morselli et al. 1978; Rane and Wilson 1976).

Furthermore, significant differences may been seen among children of different ages. Infants, children, and adolescents are not a homogenous group in terms of their drug disposition patterns (Morselli, 1977; Morselli and Pippenger 1982).

Evidence suggesting more rapid disposition of drugs in children, for studied agents, is limited to reports of smaller concentration-to-dose ratios and, in some instances, shorter plasma half-lives. Although there are several possible explanations for the more rapid disposition of drugs, more rapid hepatic metabolism in children and adolescents is usually accepted as the major mechanism. There are, however, many other factors that can affect serum drug concentrations, of which some are age-dependent.

DEVELOPMENTAL FACTORS AFFECTING SERUM DRUG CONCENTRATIONS

Bioavailability (Including Absorption)

Systemic bioavailability is of major importance in determining plasma concentrations and pharmacological effects for orally administered drugs. Systemic bioavailability is a function of gastrointestinal absorption and of the extent of hepatic extraction and metabolism of the drug during its "first pass" through the liver via the portal circulation. Decrease in gastrointestinal absorption or increase in first-pass hepatic metabolism will reduce plasma levels and increase dosage requirements. There are no data indicating a generally reduced absorption of orally administered drugs in older infants and children, but more rapid absorption has been observed for certain drugs in young children. Rapid absorption may result in higher peak levels, but does not affect average steady-state concentrations. More frequent administration of smaller doses to children has been recommended to minimize peak-to-valley fluctuations.

Volume of Distribution

After absorption, drugs are distributed or diluted into the intravascular and extravascular compartments. The larger the apparent volume of distribution (V_d), the smaller will be the plasma drug concentration (C_p) after any given dose (D): $C_p = D/V_d$. The relative proportion of total body water and extracellular water changes with age. In the newborn, total and extracellular body water are about 75 and 40 percent of body weight, respectively, compared to 40 and 20 percent in adults (Briis-Hansen 1961). The transition from the newborn to the adult pattern is a gradual one. For drugs that are primarily distributed in the body water (such as lithium), children would be expected to have larger volumes of distributions and proportionately lower concentrations.

Dose adjustments based on surface area rather than weight have been recommended for children because surface area correlates better with extracellular water, as well as with renal and hepatic blood flow. Although helpful, dosage estimates based on surface area may still underestimate dosage requirements.

Highly lipophilic drugs, such as most antipsychotic and antidepressant agents, have volumes of distribution greatly in excess of the total body water, and demonstrate lower plasma concentrations in children than adults after the same weight-adjusted doses (Rivera-Calimlim 1982). Since age-related changes in body water of the magnitude described are unlikely to affect significantly the volume of distribution of such hydrophobic drugs, other mechanisms must explain the low plasma concentrations of these lipophilic drugs in children.

Children are known to carry more adipose tissue per body weight, but this also appears to be a small factor. In the presence of a constant clearance rate, the plasma elimination half-life will be directly proportional to the volume of distribution:

$$V_d = \frac{T_{1/2} \times Cl}{0.693}$$

Since children have been reported to manifest shorter plasma elimination half-lives for a number of drugs, a greater volume of distribution cannot be the major factor in producing the relatively low plasma levels after administration of a given dosage of a lipophilic psychotropic agent.

Metabolism

Increased metabolic clearance is the most frequently suggested and most widely accepted explanation for the relatively higher dose requirements in children. Drug biotransformation by the liver is very rapid and efficient in children, and is probably the major mechanism for the increased metabolic clearance of psychotropic and other lipophilic drugs in childhood. Hepatic metabolic capacity is high in infancy, gradually declines with age, decreases sometimes abruptly and unpredictably around the onset of puberty, and reaches adult levels during adolescence. For example, the model drugs phenylbutazone and antipyrene are both metabolized by hepatic mixed-function oxidases, and show plasma half-lives in children that are about half those found in normal adults (Alvarez et al. 1975).

In general, metabolic pathways for many drugs appear to mature by about 3 to 6 months. Rates of drug metabolism are maximal during infancy and early childhood (1 to 5 years), and tend to be about twice those of adults during prepuberty (6 to 10 years), gradually declining to adult values by about 15 years of age (Morselli 1977; Morselli and Pippenger 1982). As a consequence, proportionately larger weight-adjusted doses are generally required in children to achieve therapeutic plasma concentrations.

The basis for the increased hepatic metabolism of drugs in children is not fully established, but a relatively larger hepatic mass (in proportion to body weight) has been postulated as an explanation. The relative size of the liver is greatest in infancy, about 30 percent greater in the 6-year-old than in the adult, and declines gradually until puberty (Alvarez et al. 1975).

Competition by gonadal hormones for hepatic drug-metabolizing enzymes has been suggested to explain the transiently decreased drug dosage requirement commonly found during adolescence (Morselli and Pippenger 1982). Although a change toward adult disposition rate occurs at around the onset of puberty, the exact time is variable and unpredictable. Thus more frequent measurement of plasma levels where appropriate, more careful clinical monitoring, and more flexible dose adjustment are indicated during this stage of development.

Most drugs are eliminated to a varying degree by hepatic and renal mechanisms. Drugs cleared by the liver are metabolized by various enzymatic pathways that are under genetic control and that may show different age-dependency in their development. Thus observations relating to one drug should only be extrapolated to as-yet-unstudied compounds with considerable caution.

Other Factors Affecting Serum Drug Concentrations

Kidney function, unlike liver metabolism, approaches adult levels during infancy. Renal development is probably not an important factor in age-related differences in drug disposition of most psychotropic drugs, with the possible exception of lithium.

Changes in protein binding can influence the clearance of highly bound drugs, as well as the pharmacological activity manifest at any given total drug concentration in plasma. Although reduced protein binding of some drugs occurs in neonates, a developmental difference in protein binding during childhood does not appear to be an important factor in healthy children.

In addition to the importance of developmental aspects of drug disposition, it is important to recognize other factors that may significantly affect drug disposition. Genetic influences on drug kinetics can be greater than those attributed to age. Intercurrent illness can affect renal and hepatic elimination of drugs, change volumes of distribution, and alter binding of some drugs to plasma proteins. Polypharmacy, a feature of some common psychiatric and neurological drug treatments, may be responsible for drug interactions that alter plasma concentrations and dose requirements. Noncompliance (nonadherence to the prescribed treatment) rather than biological variables can, in some instances, be the explanation of low plasma concentrations.

DISPOSITION OF SPECIFIC DRUGS DURING DEVELOPMENT

In addition to these general factors that interact to influence drug disposition during development, certain drug-specific factors contribute to age-related differences in drug serum levels, clinical therapeutic effects, and adverse responses.

Neuroleptic Drugs

The limited data on the phenothiazine and butyrophenone antipsychotic drugs suggest that their disposition is more rapid in children. Both of these classes of drugs undergo extensive biotransformation in the liver. As with many other drugs, the evidence is only indirect because systematic kinetic studies in children are not available. Rivera-Calimlim and colleagues noted that comparable doses of chlorpromazine produce lower plasma concentrations in children than in adults (Rivera-Calimlim 1982; Rivera-Calimlim et al. 1979) (Table 1). Children also demonstrate declining plasma concentrations over time while on a constant dose, suggesting autoinduction of hepatic enzymes by chlorpromazine.

Morselli and colleagues reported very similar findings in children receiving haloperidol (Morselli et al. 1979, 1982), and described a continuous correlation between age and plasma level-to-dose ratios consistent with a gradual reduction in disposition rate during development (Figure 1). Neither of these investigations excluded less efficient absorption as an explanation for the lower concentrations, but there is no reason to suspect that as a likely mechanism.

The foregoing data on disposition of neuroleptics in children should be considered in the context of possible differences in the dose-

Table 1. Developmental Pharmacokinetic Change: Chlorpromazine

Dose (mg/kg)	Plasma chlorpromazine (ng/ml)	
	Children (N)	Adults (N)
0.8–3.0	8.0 ± 2.3 (10)	16.6 ± 4.3 (6)
3.1–6.0	13.5 ± 2.7 (4)*	43.5 ± 7.2 (14)
6.1–11.0	20.3 ± 2.3 (4)*	73.6 ± 11.0 (15)

Note. At comparable doses, chlorpromazine produces a lower plasma concentration in children than in adults. Values are means ± SEM (N). Data reproduced with permission from Rivera-Calimlim et al. (1979).

*Compared to adult values, $p < .01$ by Student's t-test.

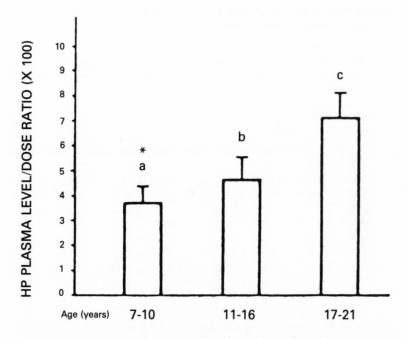

Figure 1. Developmental pharmacokinetic change: haloperidol. The plasma
level (adjusted for dosage) of haloperidol (HP) increases with
age. Figure reprinted with permission from Morselli et al. (1979).
* $p < .01$ in comparison with 17- to 21-year-olds.

response (or blood level-response) curves for childhood illnesses treated
with antipsychotic drugs. Target plasma concentrations optimal for
treatment of autistic disorder, Tourette's disorder, or childhood schizophrenia may differ from one another as well from those suggested
for management of psychoses in adults. For example, in childhood,
tics responded to haloperidol concentrations of 1 to 3 ng/ml, and
psychoses to 6 to 10 ng/ml; significant side effects were common at
concentrations above 10 ng/ml (Morselli et al. 1979, 1982). In contrast, a therapeutic range of about 8 to 18 ng/ml of haloperidol has
been suggested for adult patients with acute psychoses (Magliozzi
et al. 1981). Children appeared both to respond and to show side
effects at lower concentrations of chlorpromazine than did adults
(Rivera-Calimlim et al. 1979).

Tricyclic Antidepressant Drugs

Relatively little information is available regarding the disposition of the tricyclic antidepressant drugs in children. Since the tricyclics undergo extensive biotransformation in the liver, it would be expected that they too are metabolized more rapidly in children. The limited data available suggest that this is the case. Enuretic children treated with clomipramine were reported to show plasma level-to-dose ratios for the parent compound that increase with age (Dugas and Zarifian 1980). This same study also indicated shorter plasma half-lives and more rapid total body clearance than reported in adults.

For treatment of affective disorders in children, similar findings have been reported for the secondary amine nortriptyline (Morselli et al. 1978) (Figure 2). More rapid demethylation of imipramine, a tertiary amine tricyclic, to desipramine has also been described (Potter et al. 1982).

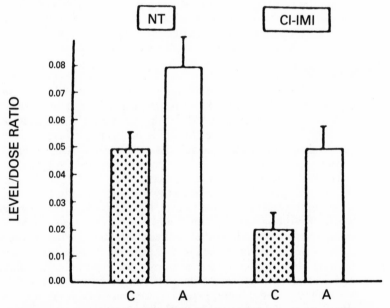

Figure 2. Developmental pharmacokinetic change: tricyclic antidepressants. Plasma levels (adjusted for dosage) of nortriptyline (NT) and chlomipramine (Cl-IMI) in children (C), aged 5 to 15 years, and adults (A), aged 18 to 55 years. Figure reprinted with permission from Morselli et al. (1978).

The manner in which this information should be translated into clinical therapeutic decision making is unclear. Optimal plasma concentrations for treatment of depression in adults are still somewhat controversial (American Psychiatric Association Task Force on the Use of Laboratory Tests in Psychiatry 1985). Even less is known about therapeutic ranges in childhood depression or the other tricyclic-responsive childhood syndromes.

An optimal therapeutic "window" of 20 to 60 ng/ml for clomipramine (Dugas and Zarifian 1980) and a threshold concentration of 80 ng/ml for the sum of imipramine plus desipramine have been correlated with successful treatment of enuresis in children (Fernadez de Gattra et al. 1984). These plasma concentrations are considerably below those that have been recommended for treatment of major depression in adults.

In children who fail to respond to tricyclic antidepressants, and in whom noncompliance is excluded, the possibility of low plasma concentrations due to rapid disposition should be considered. Although measurement of plasma concentrations may be helpful in such instances, the data should be used only in the broadest sense (e.g., to identify extremely low concentrations).

Psychostimulants

Unlike other agents considered in this review, most of the published data on the disposition of psychostimulants in humans relates to children (Gualtieri et al. 1984; Hungund et al. 1979; Shaywitz et al. 1982). Methylphenidate (MPH) is probably the best studied of the drugs used to treat attention deficit-hyperactivity disorder.

Methylphenidate therapy is somewhat distinctive in that dosing intervals are, in usual practice, very long relative to its half-life. Since the terminal plasma half-life of methylphenidate is only 1 to 2 hours (Hungund et al. 1979; Shaywitz et al. 1982), and the drug is generally administered only once or sometimes twice a day, steady-state concentrations are not achieved in ordinary clinical use. Plasma concentrations are, by intent, generally negligible by bedtime and certainly prior to administration of the morning dose. For this reason, plasma half-lives are less important than volume of distribution and bioavailability in determining plasma concentrations during the period shortly after administration of methylphenidate. Plasma half-lives of methylphenidate actually show relatively little individual variation. However, there is moderate intraindividual and considerable interindividual variation in plasma concentrations after equivalent doses, which may be a consequence of the relatively poor bioavailability

(17 to 53 percent) of methylphenidate (Hungund et al. 1979; Shay-witz et al. 1982).

There are few data comparing methylphenidate disposition in children and adults. In a study that showed no significant correlation between plasma levels and age in children receiving the same weight-adjusted dose, there was a suggestion that children might eliminate methylphenidate more rapidly than adults (Gualtieri et al. 1984). Hepatic microsomal enzymes appear to be less important than esterases for the elimination of methylphenidate in humans. Thus age-dependent disposition patterns described for other drugs may not apply to methylphenidate.

Correlation of concentrations of methylphenidate with clinical measures is controversial; therefore, a role for therapeutic monitoring of psychostimulants is not established. Current analytical methods for assaying the low plasma concentrations of this drug are not simple. However, in view of the very short half-life and unusual dosing patterns of methylphenidate, an appropriately timed drug measurement could be expected to provide an all-or-nothing answer regarding current compliance in the nonresponding patient.

Benzodiazepines

The benzodiazepines comprise a large and growing class of drugs that have hypnotic, antianxiety, and antiepileptic properties. Developmental pharmacokinetic data on benzodiazepines are largely limited to diazepam, for which there is convincing evidence of more rapid disposition in the children. Morselli et al. (1978) described the age-dependency of half-life and plasma level-to-dose relationships for diazepam (Table 2).

Table 2. Developmental Pharmacokinetic Change: Diazepam

Age group	Apparent half-life	Apparent V_d(l/kg)	Relative clearance (ml/h/kg)
Premature	75.3 ± 35.5	1.8 ± 0.3	27.4 ± 8.9
Full-term newborns	31.0 ± 2.2	—	—
Infants	10.6 ± 2	1.3 ± 0.2	98.5 ± 13.8
Children	17.3 ± 3	2.6 ± 0.5	102.1 ± 9.7
Adults	24.1 ± 5	2.3 ± 0.3	66.7 ± 5.4

Note. Pharmacokinetic parameters of diazepam in different age groups. Data reproduced with permission from Morselli et al. (1978).

The various benzodiazepines differ in their rate of elimination and in their metabolic pathways. They are variously biotransformed in the liver by N-demethylation, ring and aliphatic hydroxylation, conjugation, and by combinations of these reactions (Greenblatt et al. 1983). Except for conjugation, these processes require the actions of liver microsomal enzymes. Diazepam, for example, is N-demethylated to an active metabolite, desmethyldiazepam. Desmethyldiazepam is hydroxylated to yield oxazepam, also active, and cleared by the kidneys as a glucuronide conjugate. More rapid hydroxylation may be characteristic of diazepam disposition in children (Morselli et al. 1978). On the other hand, oxazepam and lorazepam are conjugated without prior hepatic transformation, and so are not dependent on hepatic microsomal mixed-function oxidases for their elimination. Thus it is unlikely that all benzodiazepines, despite their similar pharmacological properties, have their disposition affected by age (or other factors) to the same extent or in an identical manner.

Lithium

Lithium is almost entirely dependent on renal mechanisms for its elimination, and developmental influences on hepatic drug biotransformation are not relevant in explaining the possible developmental changes in the disposition of lithium.

Children have a higher glomerular filtration rate than adults, and are assumed to have a higher renal clearance of many drugs, including lithium (Jefferson 1982; Weller et al. 1986). Therefore higher doses have been proposed for this age group (Popper 1985). Weller et al. (1986), describing a dosing regimen for prepubertal children based on body weight, reported relatively few side effects of lithium at the standard adult therapeutic dose range (i.e., 900 to 1,800 mg/day). However, because lithium has a narrow therapeutic index, and little is known about its use and effects in children, caution and frequent monitoring of serum concentrations are recommended.

Antiepileptic Drugs

More pharmacokinetic information is available regarding this therapeutic class of drugs than for other agents used in psychiatry (Woodbury et al. 1982). This is undoubtedly a consequence of the widely accepted utilization of therapeutic drug monitoring of these drugs. With the possible exception of valproic acid (for which the data are unclear), children appear to dispose of the antiepileptic drugs at a more rapid rate and to require relatively higher (mg/kg) doses than adults to achieve therapeutic plasma concentrations (Battino et al. 1980, 1983; Bertrilson et al. 1980; Booker 1982; Garretson and

Dayton 1970; Maynert 1982; Morselli and Boss 1982; Morselli and Pippenger 1982; Svensmark and Buchtal 1964; Wilson et al. 1976; Woodbury 1982; Woodbury et al. 1982). Although decreased absorption, a larger volume of distribution, decreased protein binding, and increased metabolic clearance are all possible explanations of the lower plasma concentrations, the last is the commonly accepted mechanism. Decreased protein binding (which would affect total hepatic clearance) has been well documented for several drugs in the newborn, but does not appear to be important after early infancy.

The transition from childhood to adult disposition patterns for the antiepileptic drugs is a gradual one, culminating around adolescence, when dosage requirements can relatively abruptly and unpredictably decrease. Since presentation of side effects can be subtle in school-age children, more frequent monitoring of plasma drug concentrations is advisable for this age group (Morselli and Pippenger 1982). Current methods for analysis of antiepileptic drugs, especially immunoassays, are simple and rapid to perform and are increasingly available. The clinical significance of antiepileptic drug concentrations is reasonably well established for most commonly employed agents. Thus there is no reason for complete reliance on generalized age-adjusted dosing formulas.

Phenytoin (Dilantin), which has been well studied in children, demonstrates lower serum concentration-to-dose ratios and a shorter apparent plasma elimination half-life in children (Garretson and Dayton 1970; Morselli and Boss 1982; Woodbury 1982; Woodbury et al. 1982). Thus larger weight-adjusted doses have been recommended for younger children (Woodbury 1982; Woodbury et al. 1982). However, as a cautionary note, it should be remembered that, in children and adults, phenytoin disposition follows nonlinear, or capacity-limited, kinetics (Woodbury 1982). Thus relatively modest dosage increments can yield more substantial increases in plasma concentrations. For the same reason, phenytoin is particularly sensitive to interaction with drugs that inhibit or compete for hydroxylation in the liver, which is the major route for phenytoin disposition.

Age is only one of many factors that affect the disposition of phenytoin during childhood. Childhood illnesses such as hepatitis and glomerulonephritis, which can alter renal and hepatic function, may affect the disposition of phenytoin. Renal disease is also associated with impaired binding of phenytoin to plasma proteins, which not only alters its clearance but also increases the concentration of free or active drug associated with any given total level. Children as well as adults may be genetically "slow hydroxylaters"; therefore a subgroup of the pediatric population may have lower relative dosage requirements.

Phenobarbital, like phenytoin, yields lower plasma level-to-dose ratios in children compared to adults (Booker, 1982; Maynert 1982; Morselli 1977; Svensmark and Buchtal 1964). Weight-adjusted dosages of approximately 2 and 1.5 times the usual adult doses have been recommended for younger and older children, respectively (Booker 1982). Although phenobarbital generally has an elimination half-life of over 90 hours in adults, values of less than 50 hours have been reported in children; there is, however, considerable overlap between age groups (Garretson and Dayton 1970). In contrast to phenytoin, excretion of unchanged drug by the kidneys is a significant route of elimination for phenobarbital. Thus a somewhat higher glomerular filtration rate in children may, along with a greater hepatic metabolism capacity, contribute to the higher clearance rate observed in children. Phenobarbital can induce its own metabolism, adding an additional element of uncertainty to the prediction of plasma concentration from dosage. Fortunately, measurements of plasma concentrations of phenobarbital are readily available in most medical environments.

Carbamazepine (Tegretol) therapy is complicated by the ability of this drug to induce its own metabolism (Bertrilson et al. 1980; Morselli and Boss 1982). As a consequence of autoinduction of hepatic enzymes, steady-state plasma concentrations tend to decrease over time; upward dosage adjustments of carbamazepine may be required.

More rapid elimination of carbamazepine by children has been well documented. In a study of 326 chronically treated epileptics, Battino et al. (1983) reported that plasma level-to-dose ratios increased linearly with age (Figure 3), reaching a plateau at approximately age 19; adult values were essentially achieved by the age of 15. Significant differences in mean level-to-dose ratios were found for the various age groups of 1 to 4, 4 to 10, and 10 to 16 years, consistent with Morselli's (1977) contention that infants, children, and adolescents cannot be considered a homogeneous group in terms of their drug disposition patterns. Patients receiving concurrent therapy with phenytoin or phenobarbital had lower ratios in this study, presumably a consequence of enzyme induction. In contrast to adults, Battino and colleagues found no significant correlation between plasma concentrations of carbamazepine and weight-adjusted dose in the pediatric population. Thus, even if age-related changes are taken into account, interindividual differences in carbamazepine disposition are

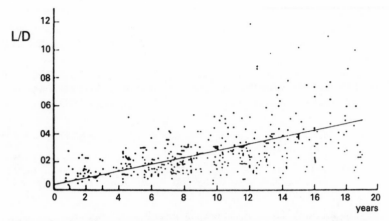

Figure 3. Developmental pharmacokinetic change: carbamazepine. Plasma level-to-dose ratios of carbamazepine in 207 children and adolescents (392 subjects, $b = 19.504$, $a = 88.046$, $df = 319$, $F_{regr} = 137$, $p < .001$). Figure reprinted with permission from Battino et al. (1980).

sufficiently great that dosage based on weight alone will be a poor predictor of plasma concentrations in children.

SUMMARY

A change in drug disposition during development is one of several important factors to consider in the management of drug therapy of children. There is good evidence that administration of comparable dosages of many drugs (including agents commonly used in psychiatry) result in lower plasma concentrations in children than in adults, and that more rapid metabolic disposition is the probable mechanism.

With children, it is often necessary to use weight-adjusted doses that are 50 to 100 percent greater than recommended adult doses.

The rapid rate of drug disposition gradually declines throughout childhood, declines sometimes abruptly around puberty, and generally reaches adult levels by mid to late adolescence. More careful clinical follow-up and drug concentration monitoring and more flexible dose adjustment are indicated during this stage of development.

Bioavailability, heredity, and a variety of normal and pathophysiological processes may influence drug kinetics and produce interindividual variations in drug disposition among children of the same age. These individual differences in drug disposition can be significant and should be taken into clinical consideration.

REFERENCES

Alvarez AP, Kapelner S, Sassa S, et al: Drug metabolism in normal children, lead poisoned children and normal adults. Clin Pharmacol Ther 17:179–183, 1975

American Psychiatric Association Task Force on the Use of Laboratory Tests in Psychiatry: Tricyclic antidepressants: blood level measurements and clinical outcome. Am J Psychiatry 142:155–162, 1985

Battino D, Boss L, Croci D: Carbamazepine plasma levels in children and adults: influence of age, dose and associated therapy. Ther Drug Monit 2:315–322, 1980

Battino D, Avanzlni G, Boss L: Plasma levels of primidone and its metabolite phenobarbital: effect of age and associated therapy. Ther Drug Monit 4:73–80, 1983

Bertrilson L, Hujer B, Gunnel-Tybring E, et al: Autoinduction of carbamazepine metabolism in children examined by a stable isotope technique. Clin Pharmacol Ther 27:83–88, 1980

Booker HE: Phenobarbital: relationship of plasma concentration to seizure control, in Antiepileptic Drugs, 2nd ed. Edited by Woodbury DM, Penry JK, Pippenger CE. New York, Raven Press, 1982

Briant RH: An introduction to clinical pharmacology, in Pediatric Psychopharmacology: The Use of Behavior Modifying Drugs in Children. Edited by Werry JS. New York, Brunner/Mazel, 1978, pp 3–28

Briis-Hansen B: Body water compartments in children: changes during growth and related changes in body composition. Pediatrics 28:169–181, 1961

Dugas M, Zarifian E: Preliminary observations of the significance of monitoring tricyclic antidepressant levels in the pediatric patient. Ther Drug Monit 2:307–314, 1980

Fernadez de Gattra M, Garcia MJ, Acfosta A: Monitoring of serum levels of imipramine and desipramine and individualization of dose in enuretic children. Ther Drug Monit 6:438–443, 1984

Garretson LK, Dayton PG: Disappearance of phenobarbital and diphenylhydantoin from serum of children. Clin Pharmacol Ther 11:674–679, 1970

Gibaldi M: Biopharmaceutics and Clinical Pharmacokinetics, 3rd ed. Philadelphia, Lea & Febiger, 1984, pp 206–215

Greenblatt DJ, Shader RJ, Abernathy DR: Current status of benzodiazepines. N Engl J Med 309:354–358, 1983

Gualtieri CT, Hicks RE, Patrick K, et al: Clinical correlates of methylphenidate blood levels. Ther Drug Monit 6:379–392, 1984

Hungund BL, Perel JM, Hurwick MJ, et al: Pharmacokinetics of methylphenidate in hyperkinetic children. Br J Clin Pharmacol 8:571–576, 1979

Jefferson JW: The use of lithium in childhood and adolescence: an overview. J Clin Psychiatry 43:174–177, 1982

Magliozzi JR, Hollister LE, Arnold KV, et al: Relationship of serum haloperidol levels to clinical response in schizophrenic patients. Am J Psychiatry 38:365–367, 1981

Maynert EW: Phenobarbital absorption, distribution and excretion, in Antiepileptic Drugs, 2nd ed. Edited by Woodbury DM, Penry JK, Pippenger CE. New York, Raven Press, 1982

Morselli PL: Drug Disposition During Development. New York, Spectrum Publications, 1977

Morselli PL, Boss L: Carbamazepine absorption, distribution and excretion, in Antiepileptic Drugs, 2nd ed. Edited by Woodbury DM, Penry JK, Pippenger CE. New York, Raven Press, 1982

Morselli PL, Pippenger CE: Drug disposition during development, in Applied Therapeutic Drug Monitoring. Washington DC, American Association of Clinical Chemistry, 1982, pp 63–70

Morselli PL, Cuche H, Zarifian E: Pharmacokinetics of psychotropic drugs in the pediatric patient, in Childhood Psychopharmacology: Current Concepts. Advances in Biological Psychiatry. Edited by Mendlewicz J, van Praag HM. Basel, S. Karger, 1978, pp 70–86

Morselli PL, Biachetti G, Durand G: Haloperidol plasma level monitoring in pediatric patients. Ther Drug Monit 1:35–46, 1979

Morselli PL, Biachetti G, Dugas M: Haloperidol plasma level monitoring in neuropsychiatric patients. Ther Drug Monit 4:51–59, 1982

Popper C: Child and adolescent psychopharmacology, in Psychiatry. Edited by Michels R, Cavenar JO, Brodie HKH, et al. Philadelphia, J.B. Lippincott Co, 1985

Potter WZ, Calil HM, Sutfin TA, et al: Active metabolites of imipramine and desipramine in man. Clin Pharmacol Ther 31:393–401, 1982

Rane A, Wilson JT: Clinical pharmacokinetics in infants and children. Clin Pharmacokinet 1:2–24, 1976

Rivera-Calimlim L: Problems in therapeutic monitoring of chlorpromazine. Ther Drug Monit 4:41–49, 1982

Rivera-Calimlim L, Griesbach PH, Perlmutter R: Plasma chlorpromazine concentrations in children with behavioral disorders and mental illness. Clin Pharmacol Ther 26:114–121, 1979

Shaywitz S, Hunt RD, Jatlow P, et al: Psychopharmacology of attention deficit disorders: pharmacokinetic, neuroendocrine and behavioral measures following acute and chronic treatment with methylphenidate. Pediatrics 69:688–694, 1982

Svensmark O, Buchtal F: Diphenylhydantoin and phenobarbital: serum levels in children. Am J Dis Child 108:82–87, 1964

Weller EB, Weller RA, Fristad MA: Lithium dosage guide for prepubertal children: preliminary report. J Am Acad Child Psychiatry 25:92–95, 1986

Wilson JT, Hojer B, Rane A: Loading and conventional dose therapy with phenytoin in children: kinetic profile of parent drug and metabolite in plasma. Clin Pharmacol Ther 20:48–58, 1976

Woodbury DM: Phenytoin absorption, distribution and excretion, in Antiepileptic Drugs, 2nd ed. Edited by Woodbury DM, Penry JK, Pippenger CE. New York, Raven Press, 1982

Woodbury DM, Penry JK, Pippenger CE (eds): Antiepileptic Drugs, 2nd ed. New York, Raven Press, 1982

Chapter 3

Developmental Pharmacodynamics

Martin H. Teicher, M.D., Ph.D.
Ross J. Baldessarini, M.D.

Chapter 3

Developmental Pharmacodynamics

Optimal treatment of children and adolescents with medicinal agents requires knowledge of developmental differences in drug responsivity. In psychiatric therapies, the developing and mature brain may respond differently to psychotropic drugs. This chapter explores the hypothesis that children and adolescents differ from adults in their sensitivity and responsiveness to psychotropic agents.

A child may respond to a drug differently from an adult due to *pharmacodynamic* factors reflecting developmental changes in neural pathways or their functions (drug-effector mechanisms). Anatomical regions and neurotransmitter systems develop at different rates and mature at different times, and the psychological and neurophysiological functions that these pathways subserve may change over time during development. Other differences may reflect what may loosely be called *pharmacokinetic* factors due to changes in drug distribution or metabolism. Adjusting the drug dosage to regulate plasma or tissue levels of a drug should minimize differences in drug responses between children and adults if pharmacokinetic factors are involved, but not if pharmacodynamic factors are responsible.

This overview provides a framework for introducing and exploring potentially important developmental pharmacodynamic differences in sensitivity and responsiveness to psychotropic drugs. It should be noted from the outset that empirical data on this topic are sparse. Few clinical studies have focused on age-related differences in drug response, even for drugs used in general medicine and pediatrics. Those that have are often hampered by the lack of normal control groups and the absence of a dose-response analysis. Surprisingly,

This work was supported in part by NIMH awards and grants MH-47370, MH-31154, and MH-36224, as well as grants from the Marion Ireland Benton Trust Fund and the William F. Milton Foundation.

there is even a relative paucity of pertinent preclinical developmental pharmacodynamic data derived from animal studies. Nevertheless, available information demonstrates prominent age-related differences in the effects of psychotropic agents, particularly in animals. This information may stimulate clinical thought and guide future research.

Terminology for Comparing Drug Effects Across Different Ages and Populations

Precise terminology is required to describe group- and age-related differences in drug effects. Figure 1 presents a classic dose-response curve. Traditionally this is a *quantal* curve indicating the percentage of subjects displaying a specific, often "all-or-none," response to a dose of drug. More commonly, *quantitative* curves are used to demonstrate the magnitude of a response as a function of drug dose. Four descriptive quantities can be extracted from this type of curve: (1) basal response; (2) maximal response; (3) the dose effective in producing a given level of response, such as a half-maximal response (ED_{50}); and (4) the steepness of the curve.

Different drugs are usually compared by reference to two of these parameters. *Potency* refers to the amount of drug required to produce a particular effect. Potency comparisons between drugs can be expressed quantitatively as the ratio of their ED_{50} values. *Efficacy*, on the other hand, is a measure of the magnitude of the drug's maximal

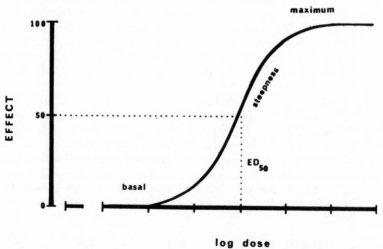

Figure 1.   Classic dose-response curve indicating change in magnitude of drug effect as a function of dose.

effect. These two concepts are distinct. Neuroleptic drugs vary widely in potency, but most appear to be indistinguishable in efficacy as indicated by their ability to treat psychotic symptoms (Baldessarini 1985). Antimicrobials, in contrast, can vary widely in the efficacy with which they treat different infections.

Potency and efficacy are typically used to describe characteristics of drugs, and are useful concepts for comparing two different drugs. Analogous concepts may also be used to compare the response of two groups of patients to the same drug. This is helpful in developmental pharmacology, where different "groups" may represent humans (or animals) at different ages. To provide a consistent vocabulary for describing group differences in drug response, we use sensitivity and responsivity regarding responses of patients (or a patient) as precise analogues to the drug descriptors potency and efficacy. *Sensitivity* refers to patients' requirement for an amount of drug to produce a desired response. *Responsivity*, in contrast, is a measure of response size or quality. Potential differences that may occur in sensitivity and responsivity between groups of patients are indicated in Figure 2. These terms and concepts are important in making group comparisons.

"Pure" differences in sensitivity alone are likely to reflect differences in drug levels in tissue due to pharmacokinetic factors, whereas true differences in responsivity often reflect pharmacodynamic differences in the underlying neural substrate or effector mechanisms.

Figure 2 also illustrates another important, but often neglected, point. If group comparisons are made in a pharmacological study using only a single dose (or narrow range of doses), it is not possible to tell whether differences in response reflect differences in responsivity or sensitivity. This problem is further complicated by the fact that many dose-response curves are multiphasic, and, at high doses, response magnitude may diminish. For example, there is some evidence that the therapeutic response to neuroleptics may diminish at doses (and blood levels) in the upper range of those in common clinical use, indicating the presence of a "therapeutic window" (Baldessarini et al. 1987a, 1987b; Teicher and Baldessarini 1985). This phenomenon is also well documented in animal studies on the locomotor effects of amphetamine. A similar phenomenon is suggested to occur in the relationship of clinical effect to plasma levels of the antidepressant nortriptyline (American Psychiatric Association Task Force on the Use of Laboratory Tests in Psychiatry 1985). Thus, if an age group shows a weak response to a fixed dose of drug in a single-dose study, they could be hyporesponsive, hyposensitive, or even hypersensitive to the drug. Only through a complete dose-

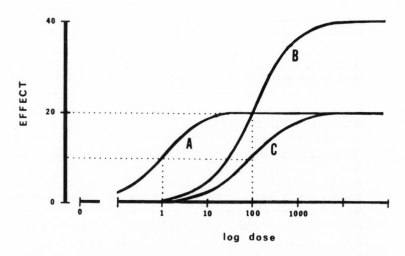

Figure 2. Classic dose-response curves demonstrating the concepts of sensitivity and responsivity. Traditionally, dose-response curves are used to compare the effects of various drugs on the same population, but they can also be used to contrast the response of different patient populations, or age groups, to the same drug. Group A is the most drug-*sensitive* group: the ED_{50} of Group A is lower than of Groups B and C. Group B is the most drug-*responsive* group: Group B members have a greater maximal response to the drug than members of Groups A and C. A clear demonstration of group differences in sensitivity and responsivity requires a dose-response study over a wide range of doses. Comparisons based on studies of a single dose, or a narrow range of doses, do not produce sufficient information to determine whether perceived group differences are due to alterations in sensitivity or responsivity.

response analysis can the nature of these differences be ascertained, even in routine clinical studies.

Clinical Observations Suggesting Age-Related Differences in Drug Action

An example that illustrates the principles just discussed is the effect of stimulant agents on children with attention deficit-hyperactivity disorder. Indeed, pediatric psychopharmacology was introduced with the report by Bradley (1937) on the behavior of a heterogeneous group of disturbed children treated with (*d,l*)amphetamine (Benzedrine). He reported that 15 of 30 children displayed striking improvement in school performance with this treatment. Many of the children became more subdued without sedation or loss of interest. Since then, many studies have supported and confirmed the "paradox" that most hyperactive children are calmed by amphetamine and excited by barbiturates, presumably opposite to the pattern expected in adults. Over several decades, much research and speculation have centered on proposed mechanisms for this supposedly paradoxical response.

Rapoport et al. (1978, 1980) were the first investigators to test rigorously the hypotheses that the sedating effect of amphetamines was either a paradoxical response of hyperactive children in comparison to normal children, or a more general developmental difference in drug response between children and adults. They compared the acute effects of a dose of *d*-amphetamine in hyperactive boys, normal boys, and college men. They found little *qualitative* difference between these groups in the effects of amphetamine on general activity, attention, or cognitive performance. Contrary to prevalent expectations, amphetamine did not increase activity in any group, and decreased reaction time and increased recall in all groups in their laboratory setting.

The effects of amphetamine on motility were more fully explored by Porrino et al. (1983) in the first naturalistic study of hyperactive children using automated activity monitoring. They found that *d*-amphetamine tended to reduce the activity level of hyperactive children, without causing sedation, during quiet periods (math class) but had a modest stimulating effect during periods of high physical activity (gym class).

It remains to be determined whether these groups display similar dose-response curves to amphetamine, as the doses selected resulted in quantitatively different group responses. Hyperactive children decreased their activity by 44 percent with *d*-amphetamine (0.5 mg/ kg), normal children experienced a 24 percent decrease at the same dose, and adults had only a 9 percent decrease at a lower dose (0.25 mg/kg) and no change in activity at the same dose (0.5 mg/kg). It is not known whether these differences indicate a slight shift in sensitivity, a group-related difference in absolute response magnitudes, or an interaction between basal response level and dose effects.

Overall, these landmark studies indicate that the overt calming effect of amphetamine is not restricted to hyperactive children, and that normal children and young adults may also be calmed in certain test settings.

In these studies, an important difference emerged between children and adults in the effects of *d*-amphetamine on mood. While this drug had a consistent euphoriant effect in adults, it produced dysphoria, irritability, and "crankiness" in both normal and hyperactive children. This age-related response difference is consistent with recent case reports of adverse behavioral side effects, including dysphoria, anxiety, and hallucinations, in some children given ordinary doses of other potent centrally active sympathomimetic agents, such as the nasal decongestants oxymetazoline (Dristan) and pseudoephedrine (Actifed and others) (Ackland 1984; Soderman et al. 1984). It is also believed that steroids produce euphoria much less frequently in children than in adults (Rapoport et al. 1980).

These findings suggest that there may be prominent developmental differences in affective response to mood-altering agents. It is possible that pharmacodynamic factors involving the developing central nervous system (CNS) are responsible. However, more detailed investigations are needed to test this hypothesis; for example, a full dose-response analysis is needed to eliminate pharmacokinetic factors.

A series of case reports suggests that carbamazepine (Tegretol) may have a much greater risk of exacerbating seizure disorders in children than adults, and that this difference may be due to the greater susceptibility of the developing brain to generalized absence seizures, which can occur as adverse effects of carbamazepine (Snead and Hosey 1985).

A potential perinatal interaction between diphenhydramine (Benadryl) and temazepam (Restoril) has been described in a case report (Kargas et al. 1985). A healthy 28-year-old woman (gravida III, para II) ingested diphenhydramine (50 mg) and, 90 minutes later, temazepam (30 mg); within 8 hours, this was followed by violent intrauterine movements and delivery of a stillborn infant. In a subsequent laboratory study, both drugs were administered to pregnant rabbits; although each drug alone was well tolerated, joint administration of both drugs produced an 81 percent fetal mortality. In the rabbits dying after delivery, seizures and marked irritability were observed. This interaction may be due to pharmacokinetic or pharmacodynamic effects. It is unknown whether this effect may occur with other benzodiazepines, histamine antagonists, or anticholinergics. This case report underscores the complexity and potential clinical importance of drug interactions, and of the possibility of age-specific pharmacological effects.

Apart from these few reports, there is little clinical literature attributing age-related differences in CNS drug response to anything other than pharmacokinetic factors. Also, we are not aware of any other empirical studies examining early developmental differences in the behavioral responses of *normal* human subjects to psychoactive drugs.

DEVELOPMENTAL DIFFERENCES IN BEHAVIORAL RESPONSES OF LABORATORY RATS TO PSYCHOACTIVE AGENTS

To explore the hypothesis that developmental pharmacodynamic differences may exist in behavioral responses to medications, we can consider preclinical studies in animals as rough guidelines to the types of pharmacodynamic differences that may occur in human development. From this vantage point, clinically relevant hypotheses can be formulated for study in humans.

Cross-Species Age Comparisons

The developing rat has been the most commonly employed laboratory test subject in developmental psychopharmacology. Unfortunately, there is no simple way to convert the age of developing rats to an approximately comparable age in humans. Such an effort is probably futile because of marked structural differences in brain regions and the rate of regional brain development between species.

The newborn rat is quite helpless (altricial). It is somewhat more motorically competent at birth than the human newborn, as it is able to locate and apprehend the mother's nipple without assistance. Righting reflexes and effective crawling develop in the first few postnatal days, and neonatal rat pups can walk with full weight support by postnatal day 10, run by day 13, and are most likely to be hyperactive when tested in isolation on day 15 (see Table 1). On the other hand, these animals are virtually deaf until about day 12 and blind until day 15, and formation of the necessary anatomical and neurophysiological substrates for these sensory functions occurs slowly. Thus 15-day-old rats are most similar to newborn children from the standpoint of visual function but, at the same time, they resemble an 8-year-old in motor development. The vast majority of research on developmental differences in psychotropic drug responses focuses on effects on motor activity in rats. Table 1 provides a set of milestones to use as a conceptual framework in which to place developmental changes in drug effects.

Amphetamine and Other Monoaminergic Stimulants

Amphetamine, an agent that indirectly stimulates the neuronal release of dopamine and norepinephrine, exerts similar activity-increasing effects in neonatal and adult rats, although these responses are longer in duration in the rat pup if the animals are tested in isolation in

Table 1. Developmental Milestones in Albino Rats

Day	Motor	Sensory	Social	Ingestive
1	Able to suckle without assistance	Olfactory, thermal, tactile present	Maternal stimulation for elimination	Suckling only
2	Scratch and righting reflexes			
3		Can orient to nest		
4	Efficient crawling			
10	Stands and walks		Leaves nest frequently	
12		Ears open		
13	Runs			
15	Hyperactive in isolation	Eyes open	Retrieval no longer possible	Suckling responsive to deprivation; starts to sample food and fluids
21	Motorically as competent as adults		Period peak playfulness	Weaning (laboratory)
30			Periadolescent period	Weaning (wild)
40			Sexual maturity	

individual cages (Campbell et al. 1969; Fibiger et al. 1970). Amphetamine administered to rat pups in other settings where they appear more aroused and behaviorally active (e.g., in a litter with the mother present) can result in decreased activity (Randall and Campbell 1976). Higher doses of amphetamine induce stereotyped behavioral responses, such as mouth movements, licking, and repetitive tongue protrusion along with diminished locomotion early in the neonatal period, similar to responses seen in adults (Lal and Sourkes 1973; McDevitt and Setler 1981).

Similar behavioral effects have also been reported following neonatal administration of L-dopa, the metabolic precursor of catecholamines, and in response to monoamine oxidase (MAO) inhibitors. Both treatments result in increased brain levels of dopamine and norepinephrine in rat pups (Kellogg and Lundborg 1972).

Thus major developmental differences in motor behavioral responses to monoaminergic stimulants are not found in the maturing rat. However, the study of agents with more selective actions on catecholamine systems have revealed prominent pharmacodynamic changes during maturation.

α-Adrenergic Agonists

Clonidine is an α-adrenergic agonist with prominent α_2 (largely presynaptic) and weaker α_1 (postsynaptic) stimulating effects in adults. The usual overall outcome is a decrease in the release of norepinephrine (by stimulation of α_2 presynaptic autoreceptors), a reduction in postsynaptic adrenergic function, and a clinical antihypertensive and sometimes sedating effect. This interesting drug has an expanding niche in neuropsychiatry, including pediatric psychiatry, with reports of its efficacy in the treatment of Tourette's disorder (Cohen et al. 1980) and attention deficit-hyperactivity disorder (Hunt et al. 1985). It is also reported to be effective in adults to aid withdrawal from opiates, alcohol, or tobacco (Glassman et al. 1984; Gold et al. 1978) and in the treatment of mania (Zubenko et al. 1984a) and neuroleptic-induced akathisia (Zubenko et al. 1984b).

Response to clonidine changes dramatically during maturation of the rat (Kellogg and Lundborg 1972; Nomura 1980). As shown in Figure 3, clonidine paradoxically stimulates activity in the rat in a dose-dependent manner during the first postnatal week. During this early period, it is about as effective in stimulating motor activity as amphetamine. At 14 days of age, clonidine produces no obvious effect on activity at any dose tested. From 20 days (about the time of weaning) into adulthood, it produces prominent dose-dependent sedation. These observations have been replicated in several labo-

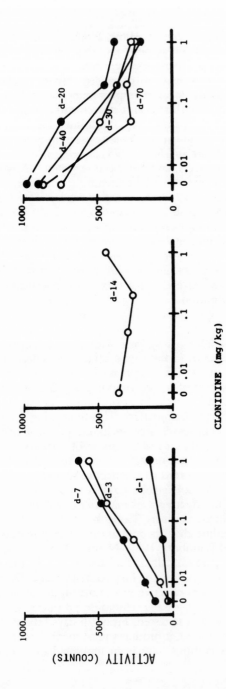

Figure 3. Developmental differences in arousal response to clonidine in rats. Effect of clonidine on arousal-associated activity levels of developing rats at age 1 week (days 1–7), age 2 weeks (day 14), and after age 3 weeks (days 20–70). Clonidine is stimulating in the neonate and becomes sedating after age 2 weeks. This figure is adapted from Nomura et al. (1980).

ratories, across a wide range of doses, and provide a compelling demonstration of a probable pharmacodynamic developmental change in responsivity to a psychotropic drug. It still needs to be ruled out that the neonate does not produce a unique stimulating metabolite of clonidine; but barring this remote possibility, this changing motor response to clonidine seems best explained as an age-related difference in drug-effector mechanisms.

There is suggestive evidence that the late emergence of sedative effects of clonidine parallels the relatively delayed and slow ontogeny of inhibitory α_2 adrenergic autoreceptors (Hartley and Seeman 1983). The mechanisms responsible for the early stimulating effect of clonidine in the newborn remain elusive, but may reflect a weak postsynaptic α_1 adrenergic agonistic action of clonidine, unopposed by the later-developing α_2 effects.

Dopamine Agonists: Postsynaptic Effects

Several studies have focused on behavioral responses of the neonatal rat to direct dopaminergic agonists, particularly R(-)apomorphine. In contrast to the effects of amphetamine or clonidine in the newborn, apomorphine does not augment arousal-associated behavior or induce stereotyped movements at high doses in the newborn rat (Kellogg and Lundborg 1972; Lal and Sourkes 1973), and is more likely to produce "stuporous" behavior (Mabry and Campbell 1977). By about 14 days of age, apomorphine produces moderate excitatory responses, and more prominent arousal is typical at later ages. A similar developmental time course has been reported for other selective dopaminergic agonists (McDevitt and Setler 1981; Reinstein et al. 1978; Shalaby and Spear 1980).

Figure 4 displays dose-response curves for 1-week-old rats, comparing the relative arousal-enhancing effects of (+)amphetamine, R(-)apomorphine, and the potent dopamine agonist R(-)N-propyl-norapomorphine (Teicher et al. 1983). In contrast to amphetamine, the selective direct dopaminergic agonist aporphines have no major effects on activity, although they may slightly augment activity at low acute doses (10 µg/kg, intraperitoneally).

These studies demonstrate that direct dopaminergic agonists do not affect low-level basal arousal in the neonate, as they do in the adult, and strongly suggest that the arousal-inducing properties of indirect catecholamine agonists such as amphetamine are likely to be mediated by norepinephrine in the neonate.

These observations might seem to suggest that the central dopamine system is not functional in neonatal rats. However, direct neurochemical studies show that metabolic turnover of dopamine is

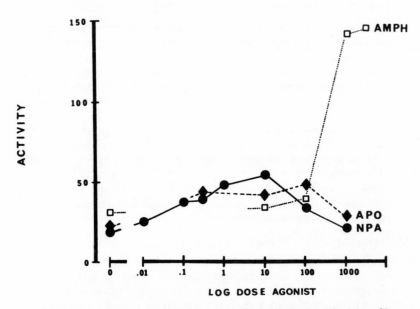

Figure 4. Effect of Catecholamine Agonists on Behavioral Activity of Rats. Dose-response comparison of effects of (+)amphetamine (AMPH), (−)apomorphine (APO), and (−)N-propylnorapomorphine (NPA) on spontaneous locomotor activity of unaroused 7- to 8-day-old rats. Dose is μg/kg of body weight. (+)Amphetamine augments basal arousal levels at doses of 1,000 to 3,000 μg/kg (1.0–3.0 mg/kg), whereas the direct dopamine agonists APO and NPA have little arousal effects in the neonates. In adult rats, all three agents produce comparable arousal effects. This figure is based on data reported by Teicher et al. (1983).

actually higher in the neonate than in the adult. This evident paradox may reflect a "ceiling" effect, by which further increments in functional activity are not possible. One way to explore this relationship is to ascertain whether agents that inhibit the dopamine system attenuate arousal behavior.

Dopamine Agonists: Presynaptic (Inhibitory) Effects

The dopamine system in some regions of mammalian forebrain is believed to be controlled homeostatically by the action of "autoreceptors" located on presynaptic dopaminergic nerve terminals, cell bodies, and dendrites. Stimulation of these receptors inhibits the production and release of additional dopamine (Roth 1979). Based on the work of Carlsson (1975), the function of dopaminergic autoreceptors can be demonstrated behaviorally by treating rats with very small doses of certain dopamine agonists. In adult rats, very low doses of these agents produce apparently antidopaminergic hypomotility, presumably related to preferential stimulation of autoreceptors, whereas 10- to 20-fold higher doses produce characteristic behavioral excitatory responses that are believed to reflect activation of postsynaptic dopaminergic receptors.

Using this paradigm, Shalaby and Spear (1980) failed to find inhibitory effects of moderate doses of apomorphine until about 28 days of age. They proposed that dopamine autoreceptor function may develop several weeks later than postsynaptic function. However, the doses of apomorphine used were rather high, and basal activity levels in their laboratory setting were so low that it would be hard to detect an inhibitory effect.

To overcome these difficulties, we evaluated the effects of a wide range of doses of apomorphine and its N-propyl congener on maternally directed locomotor responses of aroused, suckling-deprived 8-day-old rats. Such environmental manipulations produce high levels of basal activity on which to measure for behavioral inhibitory actions of test agents. As shown in Figure 5, prominent inhibitory effects of the dopaminergic agonists were found at this age following extraordinarily low doses (0.01–0.03 µg/kg, i.p.). We also found a mild excitatory effect at moderate doses that may reflect stimulation of postsynaptic receptors, as well as prominent inhibition of activity at higher doses that may reflect "overstimulation" of postsynaptic receptors.

These studies suggest that dopamine may be involved in mediating certain environmentally induced arousal responses in the neonate, and that this effect can be antagonized by autoreceptor stimulation with very low doses of dopamine-agonist aporphines (and perhaps by overstimulation or antagonism of postsynaptic elements at high doses).

In fact, neurochemical studies provided confirmation of these developmental-behavioral pharmacological hypotheses. Maternal deprivation followed by reunion of the rat pup with its mother produced the greatest increase in dopamine turnover in striatum that we have observed following environmental manipulations (Teicher, Richheld, and Baldessarini, unpublished observations).

Dopamine Antagonists

Evidence for activity of the immature dopamine system is supported by studies of dopamine receptor antagonists such as haloperidol and other antipsychotic agents. These drugs exert prominent antagonistic

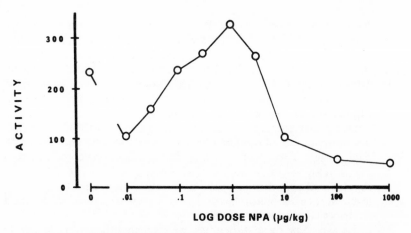

Figure 5. Effects of a dopamine agonist on behavioral activity of rats. Dose-response curve for the potent direct dopaminergic agonist (−)N-propylnorapomorphine (NPA). Rat pups at 7 to 8 days of age were tested in a highly aroused state induced by brief maternal deprivation followed by return to their anesthetized mothers. Arousal-associated behavioral activity is measured during the initial 15 seconds of reunion using a sensitive computer-interfaced vibrational activity monitor. Extremely low doses of NPA (0.01 μg/kg) significantly attenuate behavioral activity (presumably due to dopamine autoreceptor activation), whereas a 100-fold higher dose (1.0 μg/kg) produces a mild stimulatory effect. Doses beyond this level markedly inhibit behavioral arousal, possibly as a consequence of postsynaptic overstimulation. This figure is based on data reported by Teicher et al. (1983).

effects on D_2 dopamine receptors that correlate with their clinical potency (Snyder 1981). A comprehensive study of the effects of maturation and aging on the behavioral response of rats to haloperidol was conducted by Campbell and Baldessarini (1981). In these studies, 18-day-old rats were 75 times more sensitive (ED_{50} shifts) to the activity-reducing effects, 61-fold more sensitive to the sedative effects, and 18 times more sensitive to the cataleptic effects of haloperidol than adults. These changes in sensitivity were not accounted for by changes in body weight, and appear to generalize to chemically dissimilar neuroleptic agents such as perphenazine (Campbell et al., in press). Furthermore, these enormous developmental differences do not appear to be pharmacokinetic in origin because they have also been observed following direct administration of haloperidol or perphenazine into the brain, and because there were no developmental changes in tissue brain levels of these neuroleptics following systemic administration (Campbell, Baldessarini, and Teicher, unpublished observations).

Dopamine Agonists and Antagonists: Summary

Overall, the developing rat displays important changes in its response and sensitivity to agents that affect the central dopamine system. First, dopaminergic stimulation is not sufficient to augment behavioral activity dramatically until at least 2 weeks of age, but noradrenergic stimulation is sufficient to stimulate locomotor behavior even at birth. Second, environmental conditions that augment the activity and arousal-associated behavior of neonatal rats increase the metabolic turnover of dopamine. Third, inhibition of dopaminergic activity by neuroleptics or autoreceptor agonists attenuates environmentally relevant arousal responses at extraordinarily low doses in young rats.

It can be inferred that the dopamine system may be involved in mediating arousal in the preweanling rat but may be less critical than in adulthood. This hypothesis is further supported by the observation, discussed later, that neonates can tolerate nearly total destruction of their ascending dopaminergic projection systems with minimal deficits in locomotor activity. Adult rats sustaining comparable destruction are rendered akinetic and fail to eat or drink.

Hypothetically, dopaminergic "tone," or "coupling" with arousal, may be low in the rat prior to 14 days of age. It is also likely that the dopamine system is poorly or weakly regulated by homeostatic processes and can easily be overwhelmed by even modest doses of agonists or antagonists. The adrenergic system is active in moderating behavior and arousal at birth, and the dopaminergic system may be less functional until later. The clinical implications of these hypotheses will be addressed below.

Cholinergic Drugs

Agents that affect central acetylcholine systems are ubiquitous in medicine. Drugs that augment activity in these systems are being studied for potentially beneficial effects on memory and cognitive processes, and as antimanic agents. Muscarinic cholinergic antagonists are used routinely to treat Parkinson's disease, as well as dystonic and bradykinetic extrapyramidal reactions to neuroleptic drugs (Tarsy and Baldessarini 1986). Many other psychotropic drugs, notably the tricyclic antidepressants, block muscarinic receptors and produce undesired central and peripheral anticholinergic side effects.

Muscarinic cholinergic receptors emerge at still later ages than either noradrenergic or dopaminergic receptors. As a consequence, in young rats, agents that alter muscarinic activity fail to produce many of the expected cholinergic interactions with noradrenergic and dopaminergic systems seen in the adult. For example, the centrally active direct cholinomimetic muscarinic agonist pilocarpine attenuates amphetamine-induced motor activity in adult rats. Fibiger et al. (1970) found that, although amphetamine augmented arousal at all ages studied, pilocarpine failed to depress this presumably adrenergic arousal response in the rat until at least 20 days of age. Apparently, muscarinic inhibition of the adrenergic response was not seen until day 20.

Cholinergic antagonism by antimuscarinic drugs often augments arousal responses in the adult rat, but only after a sufficient degree of cholinergic maturation. For example, scopolamine stimulates locomotor activity in rats only after age 20 days (Campbell et al. 1969). Atropine accelerates locomotor activity in rats older than 30 days, but produces drowsiness and inactivity in younger animals (even in very low doses). Atropine can, however, disrupt maze learning and its retention in young rats to an extent that may exceed those effects in adults (Blozovski and Blozovski 1973).

It may be that there are regional differences in the development of central cholinergic function. Hippocampal or neocortical cholinergic systems subserving memory and learning may develop earlier than some systems subserving arousal.

These findings may be pertinent to the appearance and treatment of extrapyramidal side effects induced by neuroleptic agents in young children. Neuroleptic drugs produce cataleptic behavior in the rat as early as postnatal day 1, but the centrally active muscarinic antagonist atropine does not antagonize neuroleptic-induced catalepsy in young rats until 20 days of age (Burt et al. 1977). Although neonatal rats are unusually sensitive to the extrapyramidal effects of neuroleptic agents (Campbell and Baldessarini 1981), they are not responsive to anticholinergic antagonism of this effect (although they may be sensitive to the cognitive consequences of muscarinic blockade).

Children may be at increased risk of parkinsonism induced by neuroleptics (Keepers et al. 1983), but differences in responsiveness to anticholinergic antiparkinsonism agents have not been reported in preadolescents.

Serotonergic Drugs

Some antidepressant agents (e.g., clomipramine, trazodone, fluoxetine, zimelidine, citalopram, MAO inhibitors, L-tryptophan, and serotonin-2 antagonists such as haloperidol) may exert therapeutic effects through interactions with serotonergic systems (Baldessarini 1984, 1985). Central serotonin systems of the brain stem play a role in sleep and wakefulness and tend to suppress behavioral arousal at the forebrain level (Gerson and Baldessarini 1981). Depletion of serotonin with the competitive synthesis inhibitor p-chlorophenylalanine produces hyperactivity in the adult rat and augments the arousal response to amphetamine (Mabry and Campbell 1973). The effects of serotonin depletion do not emerge in developing rats until at least 15 days of age (Mabry and Campbell 1974).

The delayed maturation of serotonergic influences on locomotor activity may contribute to the complex behavioral effects of imipramine on developing rats. Imipramine and its active metabolite desipramine provide initial noradrenergic and serotonergic facilitation through reuptake blockade, as well as direct muscarinic and weak α_1 antagonism (Baldessarini 1983, 1985). Acute administration of imipramine to adult rats usually produces sedation. On the other hand, acute administration of large doses of imipramine to newborn and 2-week-old rats increases locomotor activity and can produce stereotyped rearing and climbing behavior (Lapin et al. 1969). By 4 weeks of age, this arousal response is lost, and sedation occurs as in the adult rat. Since noradrenergic agonists and muscarinic antagonists augment activity, it may be that the loss of imipramine-induced stimulation after 2 weeks of age is due to the delayed development of a serotonin-mediated inhibitory response. In influencing arousal-associated behaviors, the serotonin system (like the dopamine system) has a delayed ontogeny relative to the norepinephrine system.

Antidepressant agents are being used in younger children for a variety of indications (e.g., depression, enuresis, hyperactivity, phobias). It would be interesting to ascertain in the very young child whether antidepressants with strong serotonergic effects are less sedating, and whether they are comparable in efficacy to agents with more prominent noradrenergic effects. Based on the delayed ontogeny of serotonergic systems relative to noradrenergic systems, these agents are predicted to have little sedating effect in very young children and to become more sedating with maturation. The efficacy of their antidepressant properties might also change with age.

Opiate Agonists

The sensitivity to morphine analgesia is 10 times higher in 20-day-old rats than in adults, but this quickly reduces to a 3-times higher sensitivity by day 26 (Johannesson and Becker 1973). In addition, the lethality of morphine in the first 12 postpartum days in the rat is high (half-maximal lethal dose $LD_{50} = 45$ mg/kg), and decreases to an adult level (LD_{50} = 220 mg/kg) by day 32 (Kupferberg and Way 1963).

These age-related declines in pharmacological and toxicological sensitivity to an opiate in the developing rat have been thought to relate to two pharmacokinetic factors: (1) a decrease in blood-brain barrier penetration by morphine (Auguy-Valette et al. 1978) and (2) a marked increase in the rate of conjugation and plasma clearance of opiates, which occurs between 16 and 32 days of age in the rat (Kupferberg and Way 1963). On the other hand, pharmacodynamic factors may also be involved. There is a profound increase in the density of opiate receptor binding sites in the rodent brain during this same developmental period (Clendeninn et al. 1976; Kent et al. 1981).

Thus the relative contributions of pharmacokinetic and pharmacodynamic factors in producing the decrease in responsiveness and sensitivity to opiates in the maturing rat is unclear. Moreover, the relevance of these findings to human development remains to be determined.

DEVELOPMENTAL NEUROPHARMACOLOGICAL MODELS OF NEUROPSYCHIATRIC DISORDERS

Two preclinical behavioral models will be described to highlight the potential mechanisms underlying age-related changes in drug sensitivity and responsiveness. One model involves differences in drug responsivity that occur shortly before puberty. The other concerns developmental alterations in brain functions that follow irreversible destruction of dopamine systems in the developing rat. The behavioral changes and pharmacological responses observed in these models may contribute to understanding certain neuropsychiatric disorders in children.

Altered Catecholamine Sensitivity in the Periadolescent Period

Developing rats may go through a stage shortly before puberty (28 to 38 days) in which there is a transient change in their responsiveness to certain drugs. Spear and Brake (1983) reported that such periadolescent rats display diminished behavioral arousal responses to the catecholamine agonists amphetamine and cocaine, and accentuated inhibitory responses to the D_2 dopamine antagonist haloperidol. The data in Figure 6 demonstrate that these age-related differences in response magnitude are not overcome by alterations in drug dose. Therefore, pharmacokinetic differences cannot account for these effects (although there are known pharmacokinetic changes in the periadolescent years).

Spear and Brake (1983) ascribed these transient changes in responsiveness to catecholamine-stimulating and antidopaminergic agents to a putative delay in the development of mesolimbic dopamine autoreceptors. They further postulated that the later return to previous levels of response was due to a re-equilibration of pre- and postsynaptic homeostasis in limbic dopaminergic neurotransmission.

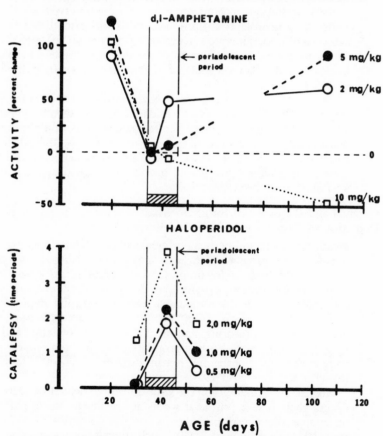

Figure 6. Changes in response to catecholamine agents during the periadolescent period. Demonstration of alterations in response to (±)amphetamine and haloperidol in periadolescent rats. During the periadolescent period, there is a decrease in behavioral activity response to amphetamine and an enhancement in cataleptic response to haloperidol. This figure is based on data reported by Spear and Brake (1983).

This explanation is questionable since selective dopaminergic agonists, such as apomorphine, produce a striking increase in locomotor activity in 35-day-old rats (Shalaby and Spear 1980), at an age when they are unresponsive to amphetamine, suggesting that the latter effect is not related to the dopamine system. Moreover, dopamine autoreceptor function emerges before this time (Teicher and Baldessarini 1985). Finally, the delayed dopamine autoreceptor hypothesis would not account adequately for the observed augmented response to neuroleptics (Campbell and Baldessarini 1981), as the presence of dopaminergic autoreceptors leads to an enhanced compensatory presynaptic activation of the dopamine system to neuroleptic blockade (Bannon and Roth 1983), and thus should diminish responsiveness.

Even though the mechanisms remain unclear, these changes in responsivity to centrally acting catecholaminergic agents in rats are striking and represent one of the few suggestions of a pharmacodynamic alteration in development. Evidence of a pharmacodynamic parallel in clinical response to catecholaminergic agents in children approaching adolescence is not known, although pharmacokinetic alterations have been identified.

Survival and Recovery of Function After Depletion of Dopamine in Neonatal Brain

Nearly complete and permanent destruction of CNS dopamine terminals of the rat during the neonatal period, using the selective neurotoxin 6-hydroxydopamine (and desipramine to protect norepinephrine neurons), provides an intriguing developmental psychobiological model. A comparable level of dopamine depletion in adult rats produces catastrophic consequences: adults became akinetic, cease to eat or drink, and die if they are not hydrated and fed by gastric intubation. With appropriate care, they can recover partially over many months, but remain extremely vulnerable to stress (Stricker and Zigmond 1976).

Neonatal rats undergoing the same dopamine-depleting treatment during their first 2 postnatal weeks are relatively unaffected and, under appropriate rearing conditions, can grow at normal rates (Bruno et al. 1984; Pearson et al. 1980). Such animals are not akinetic, but instead become hyperactive after day 15. The magnitude and duration of their hyperactivity are functions of the extent of dopamine depletion and the developmental period during which it occurs. With severe depletions, hyperactivity may not abate at all (Miller et al. 1981). Dopamine depletion prior to day 14 produces prominent hyperactivity, depletion at 20 to 23 days produces a lesser response, and later treatments are without effect or produce adult-like akinesia. Temporary inhibition of catecholamine synthesis (with alpha-methyltyrosine) during this apparently sensitive neonatal period also produces relatively persistent hyperactivity, whereas treatment of equal duration in adult rats does not.

Neonatal destruction of dopamine neurons or terminals in rats is associated with an increase in serotonin levels in the depleted brain tissues, particularly the rostral striatum. This increase occurs through collateral sprouting of serotonin terminals, as if to "replace" or "compensate" for the lost dopamine terminals (Breese et al. 1984; Stachowiak et al. 1984). This reaction is limited to the early preweaning period when the developing brain is thought to be relatively "plastic" and still anatomically adaptive. Breese and colleagues (1984) have also suggested that there is an increase in both D_1 and D_2 dopaminergic receptor function following neonatal depletions of dopamine, but that only D_2 receptor function is augmented following depletion of dopamine in adult rats.

The profoundly dissimilar responses of neonatal and adult rats to depletion of forebrain dopamine underscore major developmental changes in the brain's capacity to respond to a toxicological challenge. Since similar compensatory mechanisms may also be activated during chronic clinical treatment with dopamine antagonists, the possibility that use of these agents may alter brain development (Madsen et al. 1981) could be of clinical concern.

Shaywitz et al. (1976a, 1976b) proposed that the neonatally dopamine-depleted rat can serve as a model for the clinical syndrome of attention deficit-hyperactivity disorder. They also reported that the hyperactivity of such animals was attenuated by amphetamine and methylphenidate as in attention deficit-hyperactivity disorder (Shaywitz et al. 1981). However, the more selective direct dopamine agonists, apomorphine and bromocriptine, were not effective. Heffner and Seiden (1982) found that drugs that blocked serotonin receptors prevent amphetamine from inhibiting behavioral activity, whereas drugs that blocked dopaminergic and adrenergic receptors did not. The serotonin-releasing drug fenfluramine and the serotonin agonist quipazine also attenuated the hyperactivity of dopamine-depleted rat pups, at doses that had no effect on intact controls. These observations are consistent with the hypothesis that sprouting of serotonergic terminals in the dopamine-depleted brain region serves a compensatory function.

Breese et al. (1984) suggested that neonatal dopamine depletion can also serve as a model for some of the features of Lesch-Nyhan syndrome, a severe developmental condition associated with a disorder of purine metabolism resulting from an inborn deficiency of the enzyme hypoxanthine-guanine phosphoribosyl transferase. There is evidence that dopaminergic function in the striatum and other brain areas is reduced in patients with Lesch-Nyhan syndrome (Lloyd et al. 1981).

Administering apomorphine or L-dopa to rats following neonatal depletion of dopamine results in a syndrome characterized by self-biting, hair-pulling, and self-mutilating behaviors—all similar to the clinical Lesch-Nyhan disorder (Breese et al. 1984). The self-biting and hair-pulling behaviors were not completely reversed by halo-peridol (a relatively selective D_2 dopaminergic antagonist), whereas the thioxanthene neuroleptic cis-flupenthixol (with potent D_1 as well as D_2 dopamine receptor antagonistic activity) completely reversed these self-destructive behaviors. Apomorphine and L-dopa did not produce such a reaction in intact young rats, nor in animals depleted of dopamine in adulthood, which instead displayed only a super-sensitivity to the behavior-activating effects of these dopaminergic agents. Breese et al. (1984) speculated that neonatal dopamine de-pletion may increase the number of D_1 receptors, resulting in the expression of self-mutilatory behavior following excess stimulation. A systematic comparison of the clinical actions of various dopami-nergic antagonists has not been undertaken in Lesch-Nyhan patients.

These proposed models of clinical disorders should not be accepted uncritically. Despite the common use of the developing rat in lab-oratory-based neuropharmacological investigations, the rat is not a miniature child. Cross-species extrapolations are fraught with diffi-culty, although they can serve an important hypothesis-generating function. They may have implications regarding the prenatal and early postnatal response of the developing CNS to drugs with prom-inent neuropharmacological or neurotoxic effects, highlight the con-tribution of developmental factors to the manifestation of certain neuropsychiatric disorders, and lead to several interesting clinical hypotheses relevant to pediatric psychopharmacology.

CLINICAL IMPLICATIONS AND SPECULATION

Developmental Differences in Extrapyramidal Reactions to Neuroleptics

Preclinical laboratory data indicate that extrapyramidal responses to neuroleptic drugs emerge early in ontogeny. Rats near weaning age (approximately 21 days) are extraordinarily sensitive to the cataleptic, bradykinetic, and sedative effects of neuroleptics, and periadolescent rats (approximately 28 to 38 days) display unusually strong cataleptic reactions. These observations support the prediction that children might be more susceptible than adult patients to the extrapyramidal effects of neuroleptics.

Emerging clinical data are concordant with this prediction. Clinical observations, summarized in Figure 7, indicate that the incidence of drug-induced dystonic and bradykinetic reactions diminishes strikingly with maturation from ages 10 to 19 years to adulthood, whereas older patients show an increased risk of bradykinetic but not of dystonic reactions (Keepers et al. 1983).

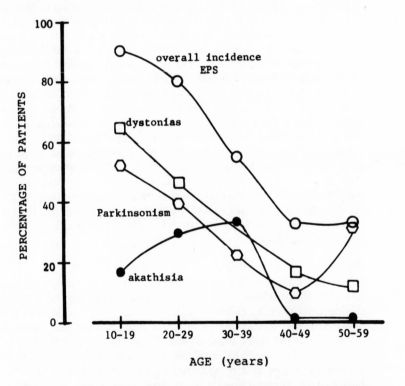

Figure 7. Age-related differences in incidence of neuroleptic-induced extrapyramidal symptoms (EPS) in humans. Age-related frequency of extrapyramidal side effects following neuroleptic drug treatment. Parkinsonism and acute dystonia follow a parallel course of decreasing incidence with maturation until 40 to 49 years, whereas akathisia follows a different time course. This figure is based on data reported by Keepers et al. (1983).

It is also noteworthy that the age-related incidence of akathisia was not found to parallel the incidence of dystonia or parkinsonism in neuroleptic-treated patients (Figure 7), suggesting that akathisia may be the consequence of a different set of neuropharmacological mechanisms. This impression is supported by recent reports that antiadrenergic agents (e.g., propranolol, clonidine) may be more useful than anticholinergics, anxiolytics, or other drugs in the treatment of neuroleptic-induced akathisia (Lipinski et al. 1984; Zubenko et al. 1984b).

It may be worth speculating further about why children do not appear more prone to the development of persistent tardive dyskinesia than adults (given that children appear to be highly susceptible to acute extrapyramidal side effects and to withdrawal dyskinesias), and why advancing age is perhaps the most influential known risk factor in the development, severity, and persistence of tardive dyskinesia (Smith and Baldessarini 1980). In addition to pharmacokinetic effects, this difference may be a consequence of age-related changes in adaptive processes. Adult rats respond to dopamine depletion (and chronic neuroleptic treatment) by developing dopaminergic D_2 receptor supersensitivity, whereas neonatal rats respond with a combination of processes that may involve sprouting of serotonergic neurons or increased sensitivity of both D_1 and D_2 dopamine receptors. A clearer understanding of the age-related differences in dopamine systems may lead to novel strategies for protecting adults against the development of tardive dyskinesia, possibly by the use of selective D_1 antagonists that are undergoing preclinical evaluation (Iorio et al. 1983).

An "Ideal" Neuroleptic Drug for Very Young Children

Given the findings on neuroleptic sensitivity reviewed above, we may speculate about which of the available neuroleptics may be safer for clinical use in young children. Unfortunately, there is no firm evidence available to indicate how adults and children may differ in sensitivity to the therapeutic action of such drugs, and there is remarkably little knowledge available to establish minimum effective neuroleptic doses at any age (Baldessarini et al. 1987a, 1987b). However, the preweanling rat is much more sensitive to bradykinetic, sedative, and cataleptic side effects of haloperidol than adults (Campbell and Baldessarini 1981). Dose-limiting forms of clinical toxicity in children may speculatively include both extrapyramidal reactions and sedation.

Current practices in pediatric psychopharmacology indicate a high rate of use of the potent neuroleptic agents, presumably on the grounds that extrapyramidal reactions can often be successfully controlled with anticholinergic medications, whereas there is no simple way to antagonize neuroleptic-induced sedation (Baldessarini 1985). The preclinical observations discussed above suggest that anticholinergic agents may be less effective against neuroleptic side effects in immature subjects, at least in very early life, when subjects may also be more susceptible to the adverse cognitive effects of muscarinic agents. However, it is not clear whether clinically significant cognitive impairment, as seen in the elderly, is associated with the use of anticholinergic agents in children.

Two neuroleptic drugs, thioridazine and clozapine, produce an atypically low incidence of extrapyramidal reactions, which may be desirable for treatment of children. However, both agents have prominent anticholinergic and sedative activity. They appear to offer little advantage over high-potency neuroleptic agents, and may even be less desirable because of the potential anticholinergic and sedative effects on cognition.

The atypical neuroleptic agent molindone, although not currently advertised for use in children under age 12, may have certain advantages. First, this agent has a relatively low incidence of dystonic and bradykinetic reactions in adults; therefore, concomitant use of an anticholinergic agent is rarely required. Akathisia is a more common adverse reaction, but young children may be somewhat less susceptible to this effect (Keepers et al. 1983). Molindone also has relatively little anticholinergic activity and is less sedating than thioridazine or clozapine. Molindone may represent a reasonable trade-off between extrapyramidal effects and strong anticholinergic and sedative properties. Furthermore, its absence of significant effects on appetite and seizure threshold make this an agent worthy of further evaluation in children. A note of caution, however, concerns the extremely short half-life of this drug in adults (approximately 90 minutes), which may require multiple daily doses, and some uncertainty regarding its antipsychotic efficacy relative to more typical neuroleptics. These presumed benefits of molindone are speculative; until empirical data are available, it would remain advisable to use more established agents in clinical treatment of children, especially very young children.

Agents Useful in Treating Attention Deficit-Hyperactivity Disorder

The rat neonatal dopamine depletion model of hyperactivity, strengthened by recent findings of serotonin sprouting in the neostriatum, suggests predictions about agents that might prove useful in the clinical treatment of attention deficit-hyperactivity disorder.

Stimulant drugs are effective in both the animal model and the clinical syndrome. More selective dopaminergic agonists such as apomorphine and bromocriptine appear to be of little value in the animal model (Shaywitz et al. 1981), possibly because they fail to stimulate serotonin receptors (Heffner and Seiden 1982). Such preclinical findings suggest that the role of serotonin as well as catecholamines in attention deficit-hyperactivity disorder needs further study.

Zametkin et al. (1985) proposed that hyperactive children might respond best to agents that affect multiple monoamine systems simultaneously, noting that the MAO inhibitors are comparable in efficacy with d-amphetamine but that imipramine has only moderate efficacy in hyperactivity (although pharmacokinetic factors might also explain these apparent differences).

Tricyclic antidepressants have been generally less effective than stimulants in controlling excessive motor behavior, but may ameliorate (or not produce) dysphoria (Garfinkel et al. 1983). It remains to be determined if the adrenergically selective tricyclic agents and agents with strong serotonergic effects are equally effective. In one study, clomipramine was significantly more effective than desipramine in reducing aggressivity and impulsivity, but there was a trend for desipramine to be more effective in improving attention in hyperactive children (Garfinkel et al. 1983). The potential association of specific monoaminergic systems with different components of the attention deficit-hyperactivity disorder may lead to more optimal treatment strategies.

The multiple monoamine hypothesis also offers an explanation for the curious clinical observation that neuroleptic agents do not necessarily interfere with the therapeutic action of stimulants in attention deficit-hyperactivity disorder. Several case reports strongly suggest that there may even be a synergistic interaction between stimulants and neuroleptics in the treatment of some children with attention deficit-hyperactivity disorder. As neuroleptic drugs tend to block many of the actions of stimulants, including their locomotor and euphoriant effects in adults, this observation seems paradoxical. However, neuroleptic agents would be expected to block stimulant actions by antagonizing dopamine-stimulating effects strongly and by partially antagonizing alpha-adrenergic effects at higher doses; serotonergic stimulation should persist. Thus such combined treatment may produce a more specific stimulation of the serotonin system (especially at S_1 serotonin receptors, because most neuroleptics block S_2 serotonergic sites), induce a mixed agonistic-antagonistic effect on the adrenergic system (possibly preventing the development of tolerance), and avoid some possible repercussions of excess dopaminergic stimulation (e.g., dysphoria, irritability).

It may turn out that, in treatment of attention deficit-hyperactivity disorder, serotonergic stimulation plays a role in reducing spontaneous activity and impulsivity and that noradrenergic stimulation enhances attention. Dopaminergic stimulation, on the other hand, may produce dysphoric side effects. The relatively nonspecific pharmacological effects of stimulants neatly fit the needs of the pediatric patient.

SUMMARY

Children, adolescents, and adults may differ in their responses to psychotropic drugs due to the developmental changes of neural systems and drug-receptor mechanisms. Age-related differences in drug responses may manifest as differences in sensitivity (amount of drug needed to achieve a given effect) or responsivity (maximum magnitude or direction of response to a drug).

Both normal children and children with attention deficit-hyperactivity disorder respond to amphetamine differently from young adults: children characteristically report dysphoric feelings with this drug, whereas adults describe euphoria. This finding cannot be explained pharmacokinetically and seems to represent a true pharmacodynamic difference.

In human laboratory studies, amphetamine attenuates motor activity in both children and young adults, but it may inhibit the activity of hyperactive children more than normal children and may exert even less inhibitory effect on young adults. Whether these trends reflect underlying age-related differences in responsivity or sensitivity remains unknown; complete clinical dose-response studies have not been conducted and pharmacokinetic factors cannot be ruled out.

Anecdotal clinical observations suggest some other possible developmental pharmacodynamic differences in drug-induced effects. Steroids may provide an example of a developmental difference in the drug-induced affective response of children and adults. There is a possibility that children may be more susceptible than adults to the adverse effect of exacerbation of seizure disorders by the anticonvulsant carbamazepine, and there is a possible diphenhydramine-temazepam interaction during the perinatal period that may increase the risk of infant mortality. These effects are not fully documented, and may be due to pharmacokinetic factors.

Animal studies provide several clear instances of age-related differences in drug response. Clonidine, an agent that stimulates inhibitory α_2 adrenoreceptors in adult rats, is a highly sedating drug in rats only after weaning (3 weeks old), whereas 2-week-old rats show little response, and younger rats are highly stimulated by this agent. This shift in response from stimulation to sedation with maturation remains to be fully explained, but probably reflects the early appearance of postsynaptic α_1 norepinephrine receptors (functioning in neurons at birth) and the slower development of presynaptic α_2 norepinephrine receptors.

Sensitivity to neuroleptic agents also changes prominently with age. Rats just prior to weaning are much more sensitive to the behavioral activity-reducing effect of neuroleptics than adult rats. These age-related sensitivity differences remain just as prominent when the drug is administered directly into the brain, bypassing differences in peripheral absorption, distribution, and elimination. The cataleptic response to neuroleptics, which can be easily observed in neonates, is not antagonized by anticholinergic drugs until after weaning, probably due to the relatively late maturation of striatal cholinergic mechanisms. It is also suspected that children are especially sensitive to certain acute extrapyramidal effects of neuroleptics and to neurotoxic effects of anticholinergic agents.

Further differences in drug sensitivity and responsivity may emerge during the periadolescent period. Rats appear then to be transiently less responsive to the stimulating effects of amphetamine or cocaine and more responsive to the cataleptic effects of haloperidol.

Finally, the consequences of neurotoxic destruction of dopamine terminals in the CNS change dramatically with age. Adult rats become akinetic, aphagic, and adipsic following nearly complete destruction of their striatal dopamine system. Neonatal rats with comparable depletions continue to suckle well, wean readily at the appropriate age, and are transiently hyperactive. Neurochemical adaptation to the early lesion, possibly involving increased development of striatal serotonergic systems, may underlie this remarkable age-related difference in response to dopamine depletion.

A great deal of additional research is needed to ascertain the scope of age-related changes in response to psychotropic drugs in humans. Such developmental neuropharmacological knowledge may provide a basis for understanding age-related differences in the effects of neuroleptics, including the incidence of their extrapyramidal side effects, and the age-dependent likelihood of recovery from withdrawal dyskinesias. Refinements in choice of specific antipsychotic and antidepressant drug treatments, selected to optimize therapeutic and side effects at different ages, might result from developmental pharmacodynamic science.

As pharmacokinetic and pharmacodynamic developmental effects are better understood, such knowledge may aid in tailoring effective therapeutic strategies for children with attention deficit-hyperactivity disorder, major depression, bipolar disorder, phobias, panic, psychosis, tic, and other disorders usually first evident in childhood, and also in the design of more optimal treatment regimens for adults.

REFERENCES

Ackland FM: Hallucinations in a child after drinking triprolidine/pseudoephedrine linctus. Lancet 1:1180, 1984

American Psychiatric Association Task Force on the Use of Laboratory Tests in Psychiatry: Tricyclic antidepressants: blood level measurements and clinical outcome: an American Psychiatric Association Task Force report. Am J Psychiatry 142:155–162, 1985

Auguy-Valette A, Cros J, Gouarderes C, et al: Morphine analgesia and cerebral opiate receptors: a developmental study. Br J Pharmacol 63:303–308, 1978

Baldessarini RJ: Biomedical Aspects of Depression and Its Treatment. Washington, DC, American Psychiatric Press, 1983

Baldessarini RJ: Treatment of depression by altering monoamine metabolism: precursors and metabolic inhibitors. Psychopharmacol Bull 20:224–239, 1984

Baldessarini RJ: Chemotherapy in Psychiatry: Principles and Practice. Cambridge, Mass, Harvard University Press, 1985

Baldessarini RJ, Cohen BM, Teicher MH: Pharmacological treatment of psychoses with neuroleptic agents, in Treatment of Acute Psychosis: Current Concepts and Controversies. Edited by Levy ST, Ninan PT. New York, Jason Aronson, 1987a (in press)

Baldessarini RJ, Cohen BM, Teicher MH: Significance of neuroleptic dose and plasma level in the pharmacological treatment of psychoses. Arch Gen Psychiatry 1987b (in press)

Bannon MJ, Roth RH: Pharmacology of mesocortical dopamine neurons. Pharmacol Rev 35:53–68, 1983

Blozovski D, Blozovski M: Effets de l'atropine sur l'exploration, l'apprentissage et l'activite electrocorticale chez le rat au cours du development. Psychopharmacologia 33:39–52, 1973

Bradley C: The behavior of children receiving Benzedrine. Am J Psychiatry 44:577–585, 1937

Breese GR, Baumeister AA, McCown TJ, et al: Behavioral differences between neonatal and adult 6-hydroxydopamine-treated rats to dopamine agonists: relevance to neurological symptoms in clinical syndromes with reduced brain dopamine. J Pharmacol Exp Ther 231:343–354, 1984

Bruno JP, Snyder AM, Stricker EM: Effect of dopamine-depleting brain lesions on suckling and weaning in rats. Behav Neurosci 98:156–161, 1984

Burt DK, Crowner ML, Hungerford SM, et al: Postnatal maturation of a cholinergic influence on neuroleptic catalepsy. Neuroscience Abstracts 3:102, 1977

Campbell A, Baldessarini RJ: Effects of maturation and aging on behavioral responses to haloperidol in the rat. Psychopharmacology 73:219–222, 1981

Campbell A, Baldessarini RJ, Teicher MH: Decreasing sensitivity to phenothiazine and butyrophenone neuroleptics given intracerebrally or systemically to developing rats. Psychopharmacology 1987 (in press)

Campbell BA, Lytle LD, Fibiger HC: Ontogeny of adrenergic arousal and cholinergic inhibitory mechanisms in the rat. Science 166:635–637, 1969

Carlsson A: Receptor-mediated control of dopamine metabolism, in Pre- and Postsynaptic Receptors. Edited by Usdin E, Bunney WE Jr. New York, Marcel Dekker, 1975, pp 49–65

Clendeninn NJ: Petraitis M, Simon EJ: Ontological development of opiate receptors in rodent brain. Brain Res 118:157–160, 1976

Cohen DJ, Detlor J, Young JG, et al: Clonidine ameliorates Gilles de la Tourette syndrome. Arch Gen Psychiatry 37:130–137, 1980

Fibiger HC, Lytle LD, Campbell BA: Cholinergic modulation of adrenergic arousal in the developing rat. J Comp Physiol Psychol 72:384–389, 1970

Garfinkel BD, Wender PH, Sloman L, et al: Tricyclic antidepressant and methylphenidate treatment of attention deficit disorder in children. J Am Acad Child Psychiatry 22:343–348, 1983

Gerson SC, Baldessarini RJ: Motor effects of serotonin in the central nervous system. Life Sci 27:1435–1451, 1980

Glassman AH, Jackson WK, Walsh BT, et al: Cigarette craving, smoking withdrawal, and clonidine. Science 226:864–866, 1984

Gold MS, Redmond DE Jr, Kleber HD: Clonidine blocks acute opiate withdrawal symptoms. Lancet 2:599–602, 1978

Hartley EJ, Seeman P: Development of receptors for dopamine and noradrenaline in rat brain. Eur J Pharmacol 91:391–397, 1983

Heffner TG, Seiden LS: Possible involvement of serotonergic neurons in the reduction of locomotor hyperactivity caused by amphetamine in neonatal rats depleted of brain dopamine. Brain Res 244:81–90, 1982

Hunt RD, Minderaa RB, Cohen DJ: Clonidine benefits children with attention deficit disorder and hyperactivity: report of a double-blind placebo-crossover therapeutic trial. J Am Acad Child Psychiatry 24:617–629, 1985

Iorio LC, Barnett A, Leitz FH, et al: SCH 23390, a potential benzazepine antipsychotic with unique interactions on dopaminergic systems. J Pharmacol Exp Ther 226:462–468, 1983

Johannesson T, Becker BA: Morphine analgesia in rats at various ages. Acta Pharmacol Toxicol (Copenh) 33:429–441, 1973

Kargas GA, Kargas SA, Bruyere HJ, et al: Perinatal mortality due to interaction of diphenhydramine and temazepam. N Engl J Med 313:1417, 1985

Keepers GA, Clappison VJ, Casey DE: Initial anticholinergic prophylaxis for acute neuroleptic induced extrapyramidal syndromes. Arch Gen Psychiatry 40:1113–1117, 1983

Kellog C, Lundborg P: Ontogenic variations in response to L-dopa and monoamine receptor-stimulating agents. Psychopharmacologia 23:187–200, 1972

Kent JL, Pert CB, Herkenham M: Ontogeny of opiate receptors in rat forebrain: visualization by in vitro autoradiography. Brain Res 254:487–504, 1981

Kupferberg NJ, Way EL: Pharmacologic basis for the increased sensitivity of the newborn rat to morphine. J Pharmacol Exp Ther 141:105–112, 1963

Lal S, Sourkes TL: Ontogeny of stereotyped behavior induced by apomorphine and amphetamine in the rat. Archives Internationales de Pharmacodynamie 202:171–182, 1973

Lapin IP, Osipova SV, Uskova NV, et al: Pharmacological effects of imipramine and desmethylimipramine in developing rats. Psychopharmacologia 14:255–265, 1969

Lipinski JF Jr, Zubenko GS, Cohen BM, et al: Propranolol in the treatment of neuroleptic induced akathisia. Am J Psychiatry 141:412–415, 1984

Lloyd KG, Hornykiewicz O. Davidson L, et al: Biochemical evidence of dysfunction of brain neurotransmitters in the Lesch-Nyhan syndrome. N Engl J Med 305:1106–1111, 1981

Mabry PD, Campbell BA: Serotonergic inhibition of catecholamine-induced behavioral arousal. Brain Res 49:381–391, 1973

Mabry PD, Campbell BA: Ontogeny of serotonergic inhibition of behavioral arousal in the rat. Journal of Comparative and Physiological Psychology 86:193–201, 1974

Mabry PD, Campbell BA: Developmental psychopharmacology, in Handbook of Psychopharmacology, Vol. 7: Principles of Behavioral Pharmacology. Edited by Iversen LL, Iversen SD, Snyder SH. New York, Plenum, 1977, pp 393–444

Madsen JR, Campbell A, Baldessarini RJ: Effects of prenatal treatment of rats with haloperidol due to altered drug distribution in neonatal brain. Neuropharmacology 20:931–939, 1981

McDevitt JT, Setler PE: Differential effects of dopamine agonists in mature and immature rats. Eur J Pharmacol 72:69–75, 1981

Miller FE, Hefner TG, Kotake C, et al: Magnitude and duration of hyperactivity following neonatal 6-hydroxydopamine is related to the extent of brain dopamine depletion. Brain Res 229:123–132, 1981

Nomura Y: The locomotor effect of clonidine and its interaction with alpha-flupenthixol or haloperidol in the developing rat. Naunyn Schmiedeberg's Arch Pharmacol 313:33–37, 1980

Pearson DE, Teicher MH, Shaywitz BA, et al: Environmental influences on body weight and behavior in developing rats after neonatal 6-hydroxydopamine. Science 290:715–717, 1980

Porrino LJ, Rapoport JL, Behar D, et al: A naturalistic assessment of the motor activity of hyperactive boys, II: stimulant drug effects. Arch Gen Psychiatry 40:688–693, 1983

Randall PK, Campbell BA: Ontogeny of behavioral arousal in rats: effect of maternal and sibling presence. J Comp Physiol Psychol 90:453–459, 1976

Rapoport J, Buchsbaum MS, Zahn TP, et al: Dextroamphetamine: cognitive and behavioral effects in normal prepubertal boys. Science 199:560–563, 1978

Rapoport J, Buchsbaum MS, Weingartner H, et al: Dextroamphetamine: its cognitive and behavioral effects in normal and hyperactive boys and normal men. Arch Gen Psychiatry 37:933–943, 1980

Reinstein DK, McClearn D, Isaacson RI: The development of responsiveness to dopaminergic agonists. Brain Res 150:216–223, 1978

Roth RH: Dopamine autoreceptors: pharmacology, function and comparison with postsynaptic dopamine receptors. Community Psychopharmacology 3:429–445, 1979

Shalaby IA, Spear LP: Psychopharmacological effects of low and high doses of apomorpine during ontogeny. Eur J Pharmacol 67:451–459, 1980

Shaywitz BA, Klopper JH, Yager RD, et al: Paradoxical response to amphetamine in developing rats treated with 6-hydroxydopamine. Nature 261:153–155, 1976a

Shaywitz BA, Yager RD, Klopper JH: Selective brain dopamine depletion in developing rats: an experimental model of minimal brain dysfunction. Science 191:305–308, 1976b

Shaywitz BA, Lipton SV, Teicher MH, et al: Effects of bromocriptine in developing rat pups after 6-hydroxydopamine. Pharmacol Biochem Behav 15:443–448, 1981

Smith JM, Baldessarini RJ: Changes in prevalence, severity, and recovery in tardive dyskinesia with age. Arch Gen Psychiatry 37:1368–1373, 1980

Snead OC, Hosey LC: Exacerbation of seizures in children by carbamazepine. N Engl J Med 313:916–921, 1985

Snyder SH: Dopamine receptors, neuroleptics and schizophrenia. Am J Psychiatry 138:460–464, 1981

Soderman P, Sahlberg D, Wiholm BE: CNS reactions to nose drops in small children. Lancet 1:573, 1984

Spear LP, Brake SC: Periadolescence: age-dependent behavior and psychopharmacological responsivity in rats. Dev Psychobiol 16:83–109, 1983

Stachowiak MK, Bruno JP, Synder AM, et al: Apparent sprouting of striatal serotonergic terminals after dopamine-depleting lesions in neonatal rats. Brain Res 291:164–167, 1984

Stricker EM, Zigmond MJ: Recovery of function following damage to central catecholamine-containing neurons: a neurochemical model for the lateral hypothalamic syndrome, in Progress in Psychobiology and Physiological Psychology, Vol. 6. Edited by Sprague JM, Epstein AN. New York, Academic Press, 1976, pp 121–188

Tarsy D, Baldessarini RJ: Clinical and pathophysiologic features of movement disorders induced by psychotherapeutic agents, in Movement Disorders. Edited by Donald A, Shah N. New York, Plenum, 1986, pp 365–389

Teicher MH, Baldessarini RJ: Selection of neuroleptic dosage. Arch Gen Psychiatry 42:636–637, 1985

Teicher MH, Sebastian S, Baldessarini RJ: Behavioral evidence for dopamine autoreceptor function in eight-day-old rats. International Society of Developmental Psychobiology, 1983

Zametkin A, Rapoport JL, Murphy DL, et al: Treatment of hyperactive children with monoamine oxidase inhibitors, 2: clinical efficacy. Arch Gen Psychiatry 42:962–966, 1985

Zubenko GS, Cohen BM, Lipinski JF Jr, et al: Clonidine in the treatment of mania and mixed bipolar disorder. Am J Psychiatry 141:1617–1618, 1984a

Zubenko GS, Cohen BM, Lipinski JF Jr, et al: Use of clonidine in treating neuroleptic-induced akathisia. Psychiatry Res 13:253–259, 1984b

Chapter 4

Developmental Neurotoxicology

Joel Herskowitz, M.D.

Chapter 4

Developmental Neurotoxicology

As infants, children, and adolescents become candidates for psychopharmacologic therapy, clinicians are giving special attention to putative long-range effects of these medical treatments on the body and the brain. This chapter will review known long-term effects of medications used throughout the fields of pediatrics, neurology, and psychiatry.

Current documentation of drug-induced biochemical and physiological changes, morphological manifestations, and behavioral symptoms will illustrate major principles of developmental neurotoxicology, and identify areas of useful clinical concern.

The agents discussed here will include commonly used medications such as anticonvulsants and antipsychotics; formerly used drugs such as thalidomide; lead and alcohol, which are not used in clinical treatment but can have profound effects on the developing nervous system; and agents such as hexachlorophene and tetracyclines, which do not primarily affect the nervous system but are developmentally toxic.

A developmental framework is useful for viewing toxic effects of drugs (Spencer and Schaumburg 1980). Six stages of development will be considered: (1) preconception, (2) pregnancy, (3) birth, (4) infancy and early childhood, (5) later childhood, and (6) adolescence (Table 1).

PRECONCEPTION

Prior to the formation of a human gamete, both sperm and egg cells are subject to toxic influences. The newborn human female already has a full collection of oocytes, which undergo further development and possible fertilization in 1 to 4 decades. During this lengthy period of vulnerability, the mutagenic effects of ionizing radiation on egg cells are well established; it would not be surprising to uncover adverse effects of chemical agents too. Cytotoxic drugs, clinically used to treat trophoblastic disease in women, have not been found

Table 1. Developmental Stages and Neurotoxic Agents

Developmental Stage	Drug	Long-Term Toxic Effect	Mechanism
Preconception	dioxin	?birth defects	?molecular damage
Pregnancy	thalidomide	somatic, neurological	protein synthesis inhibition
	tetracycline	tooth and organ discoloration	calcium binding
	alcohol	neurological, behavioral, cognitive, craniofacial, body growth	?(rule out poor care and malnutrition)
	marijuana	similar to alcohol	?(rule out poor care and malnutrition)
	trimethadione	developmental delays, craniofacial, cardiac, somatic	?
	phenytoin	developmental delays, cerebellar, craniofacial, cardiac, somatic, body growth	?
	valproic acid	spina bifida	?interference with zinc metabolism
	lithium	cardiovascular, somatic	?
	isotretinoin	brain, cardiac, facial	?
Birth	obstetric medication	alteration of parent-infant bonding	infant sedation or stimulation
Infancy	phenobarbital	cognitive, behavioral	sedation
	phenytoin	?cerebellar atrophy	postintoxication
	hexachlorophene	seizures ?neurological damage	myelin damage

Childhood	food colorings	cognitive, behavioral	?
	lead	cognitive, behavioral	enzyme inhibition
	phenobarbital	cognitive, behavioral	"disinhibition" acute oversedation in long-term use
	carbamazepine	behavioral excitation	?tricyclic-like stimulation
	phenytoin	?cerebellar atrophy	post-intoxication
	valproic acid	hepatotoxicity	?liver mitochondria enzyme inhibition
	psychostimulant	growth retardation	?
	aspirin	Reye's syndrome	?liver mitochondria enzyme inhibition
	antidepressants (tricyclic)	dental caries	anticholinergic xerostomia
	neuroleptics	dyskinesias (usually reversible) dental caries	?dopaminergic overactivity anticholinergic xerostomia
Adolescence	psychostimulant	growth suppression	growth retardation at epiphyseal closing time
	marijuana	cognitive, behavioral	oversedation
	alcohol	cognitive, behavioral	oversedation
	lithium	thyroid dysfunction	interference with TSH and synthesis of thyroxin
		skin scarring	severe acne

to exert toxic effects on gametes expressed in subsequent childhood or adult pathology (Van Thiel et al. 1970). Yet an excess of fetal loss is found among nurses with occupational exposure to the antineoplastic drugs cyclophosphamide, doxorubicin, and vincristine (separately or in combination) during the first trimester of pregnancy (Selevan et al. 1985). Toxic exposures at this early stage may result in reduced viability, or covert abortion, rather than developmental pathology.

Sperm cells, first formed during adolescence, do not have the same kind of lengthy temporal vulnerability as oocytes. Still, toxic influences on males prior to fertilization may be postulated. Proposed mechanisms for male-mediated preconceptual toxin-induced birth defects include (1) chromosome breakage in sperm cells, (2) gene sequence mutations in sperm cells, and (3) direct effects on fertilized eggs due to drugs in semen transferred to the mother through intercourse soon after fertilization (Friedman 1984).

Considerable attention has been paid to dioxin (2,3,7,8-tetra-chlorodibenzo-p-dioxin), a contaminant of the herbicide and defoliant Agent Orange used in the Vietnam War, as a possible cause of birth defects in the offspring of exposed men, but the available evidence does not support the contention that prior male exposure to Agent Orange increases the risk of having a child with a birth defect (Dan 1984; Erickson et al. 1984; Friedman 1984). If established, dioxin would be the first drug known to exert effects by this mechanism in humans.

At present, there are no established toxicological effects of drugs on sperm cells in humans. This may be partly due to the protective influence of the blood-testis barrier, a pharmacological barrier that functions similarly to the blood-brain barrier.

In animals, however, toxic exposure of sperm has demonstrated effects on offspring. Lead, ethanol, or caffeine, when ingested by males prior to mating, have been shown to influence neonatal survival, birth weight, and litter size (Soyka and Joffe 1980).

Environmental exposure to drugs or toxins prior to conception may cause alterations in somatic development or survival (viability). Lithium and the tricyclic antidepressant desipramine have been found to reduce sperm viability in vivo (Amsterdam et al. 1981; Levin et al. 1981). A variety of psychotropic drugs may alter sperm function in vitro, including neuroleptics, anticonvulsants, and propranolol (Christiansen et al. 1975; Hong et al. 1981, 1982). However, there are no demonstrated clinical effects of these drugs on rates of conception, and no agent has yet been shown to be toxic to human oocytes or sperm in a manner that results in childhood or adult pathology. Cytotoxicity at this early stage would probably appear as abortion or infertility rather than as developmental disorder.

PREGNANCY

By contrast, many drugs are known to affect intrauterine development: thalidomide, tetracyclines, certain anticonvulsants, lithium, alcohol, possibly marijuana, and many others. Drugs safe for adults may be toxic to growth during embryonic-fetal development. The province of teratology is a large and expanding area of medicine. Teratogens will be briefly reviewed with an emphasis on developmental neurotoxicology, illustrating principles of clinical treatment of children and adolescents.

In considering toxicological effects during pregnancy, it is helpful to picture the intrauterine development of the nervous system (Herskowitz and Rosman 1982; Suzuki 1980). During the third week after conception, the brain and spinal cord originate from an infolding of the neural plate. The anterior portion of this neural tube develops into the brain, and the posterior section becomes the spinal cord. Identifiable neurotransmitter-specific nuclei can be seen as early as the fourth week of gestation. The brain transforms from a smooth globular structure to a convoluted mass, as growth causes the brain to fold and form cortical gyri. Simultaneously, primitive cells adjacent to the rudimentary ventricles proliferate and migrate out toward the cortex. As axons and dendrites lengthen, myelination of nerve fibers begins during the first half of fetal life, and continues at least into adolescence and young adulthood (Yakovlev and Lecours 1967).

The first 56 days of gestation are defined as the "embryonic" period, succeeded by the "fetal" period. The teratogenic effects of various drugs and diseases, such as rubella infection or toxoplasmosis, peak in the embryonic period (Tuchmann-Duplessis 1970) and remain significant in the fetal period.

Thalidomide, an agent formerly used during pregnancy for its sedative effects, can produce profound disturbances in body growth and configuration. Some 7,000 persons were affected in the 1950s and early 1960s. The time of greatest vulnerability appears to be 35 to 50 days after the last menstrual period. The seal-limb deformity (phocomelia) is well known, but thalidomide can also produce severe adverse neurological and behavioral effects. Nearly 20 percent of 389 thalidomide victims in a study from the United Kingdom were deaf, almost 10 percent had a facial palsy, and 2 percent had epilepsy (Ouibell 1981). Five individuals (1.3 percent) were autistic, compared with a general occurrence of 0.05 percent.

Experimental work in animals suggests that thalidomide causes teratogenicity and neuropathy by interfering with ribosomal function, binding aliphatic amines that play a role in maintaining ribonucleic acid integrity (Sterman and Schaumburg 1980).

No currently used psychotropic drugs are known to inhibit protein synthesis at clinical doses, but alcohol and marijuana might cause a similar inhibition of ribosomal function.

Tetracyclines provide another illustration of drugs that can be used with relative impunity in adults, but that can have important side effects in children. Between the fifth gestational month and the eighth postnatal year, tetracyclines can cause permanent yellow or brown tooth discoloration (Rosenstein 1982). The staining was originally described in 5 percent of 300 children with cystic fibrosis treated continuously with a tetracycline for at least a year (Schwachman and Schuster 1956). The degree of staining depends on the stage of tooth formation (Moffet 1975) and the dose and duration of tetracycline therapy (Bevelander and Nakahara 1966; Grossman et al. 1971), but even short intermittent courses of tetracycline therapy produce mild discoloration that can be visualized by use of an ultraviolet light (Grossman et al. 1971; Weyman and Porteous 1963). Staining may also be influenced by different preparations of tetracycline (Moffet 1975). Tooth staining appears to be a consequence of drug binding to calcium during times of enamel formation; therefore, its main impact is observed in children whose teeth are actively developing (Lambrou et al. 1977).

In addition to enamel staining, tetracycline can cause bone to become discolored yellow, and thyroid tissues may turn brown or blue-black. The clinical significance of the bone and thyroid findings has not been established (White and Besanceney 1983).

No other antibiotics in current clinical use have been implicated in causing such effects. The finding that certain neuroleptics block calcium channels suggests a possible value in monitoring tooth color when these antipsychotic agents are used during pregnancy and childhood (Snyder and Reynolds 1985).

As with thalidomide, tetracyclines demonstrate that some pediatric toxicity may not be anticipated from animal studies or experience with a particular drug in adults.

Alcohol use during pregnancy has been suspected for several centuries to exert toxic effects on the developing fetus (Golub and Golub 1981; Hill and Kleinberg 1984). "Fetal alcohol syndrome" (Jones and Smith 1973; Lemoine et al. 1968) is characterized by three major areas of developmental abnormality: (1) prenatal and postnatal growth retardation; (2) abnormal craniofacial features, such as microcephaly and underdevelopment of midfacial structures (maxillary hypoplasia, cleft palate, micrognathia, short palpebral fissures, epicanthal folds); and (3) neurological abnormalities such as mental retardation, attentional disorders, hyperactivity, and electroencephalogram (EEG) irregularities (Hill and Kleinberg 1984).

The quantity of ingested alcohol is one important factor in determining the severity of effects. In a study that compared pregnant women who entirely or almost completely abstained with women who drank moderately or heavily (two or more drinks daily), the drinking group had more infants with low birth weight, spontaneous abortions, premature births, and infants with morphological or neurological abnormalities (Hingson et al. 1982).

Concomitant usage of other drugs may interact with alcohol in producing "fetal alcohol syndrome." A large prospective study of maternal alcoholism found that pregnant women who smoked marijuana were five times more likely than nonusers to give birth to a child with somatic, facial, and neurological features of the fetal alcohol syndrome (Hingson et al. 1982).

Alcohol and marijuana do not appear to be the exclusive determinants in producing the so-called fetal alcohol syndrome. A lack of diagnostic prenatal X-rays and a weight gain of less than 5 pounds during the pregnancy were also associated. Low weight gain might be the result of poor nutrition, infectious disease, depression, inadequate prenatal care, or metabolic disorder such as diabetes mellitus or hyperthyroidism.

Substance abuse, malnutrition, and poverty may independently or interactively contribute to the appearance of this drug-induced developmental disorder.

Anatomical studies in animals have demonstrated a variety of effects of alcohol on the developing nervous system not attributable to malnutrition. Rats exposed to ethanol during pregnancy, and through the period of lactation, show (1) reduced brain weight, (2) diminished thickness of the cerebral cortex, and (3) decreased extent of some dendrites (Schapiro et al. 1984). Myelin formation, particularly postnatally, can be impaired by alcohol exposure.

At the molecular level, alcohol has numerous cellular effects throughout the body. Specific mechanisms have not yet been fully elucidated. Alcohol alters properties of bilayered phospholipid membranes, changes cation movements including calcium, and modifies the release of many neurotransmitters and neuromodulators (Melgaard 1983).

Effects of intrauterine alcohol exposure on the behavior and learning of school-aged children have been demonstrated. Among 87 children in a learning disabilities clinic, 15 children had a history of heavy maternal drinking during pregnancy (Shaywitz et al. 1980). These children, who manifested attention deficit-hyperactivity disorder, presented a spectrum of dysmorphic features consistent with the fetal alcohol syndrome.

Fetal exposure to alcohol, by itself or in conjunction with other toxins, may lead to enduring anatomical alterations (microcephaly, somatic dysmorphism) and behavioral changes (hyperactivity, attentional disorder) in humans. Current studies have not defined a low level of alcohol ingestion that may be considered neurologically or somatically safe.

Marijuana is the most widely used illicit drug in the United States (Nicholi 1983), particularly among adolescents and children. The main psychoactive ingredient is delta-9-tetrahydrocannabinol, but different samples may contain variable cannabinoid contents and perhaps contaminants such as bacteria, the herbicide paraquat, the mold aspergillus, and other drugs such as phencyclidine ("angel dust"), which complicate the interpretation of clinical studies of use of "street drugs."

Of 1,690 inner-city mothers, 14 percent gave self-reports of marijuana use during pregnancy (Hingson et al. 1982), and their infants were 105 g (3.5 oz) lighter than infants of nonusers. A small study of 25 women who used cannabis during pregnancy did not find an increased incidence of minor physical anomalies among the children (O'Connell and Fried 1984).

Since the clinical symptoms of the fetal alcohol syndrome are five times more likely in children of mothers who smoke marijuana during pregnancy, the "alcohol" label on the syndrome is perhaps questionable. The roles of other chemical toxins such as marijuana and of interacting socioenvironmental influences are not adequately emphasized in this designation.

Multiple toxin exposure, especially in illegal street samples, constitutes a culturally new source of danger. Physical, cognitive, and behavioral consequences of marijuana use during pregnancy, including attention deficit-hyperactivity disorder, are being reported, but remain to be distinguished from effects of other drugs.

Anticonvulsant drugs, over the past decade, have been recognized to produce major malformations, including abnormalities of the central nervous system (Table 2). High infant morbidity is associated with maternal seizures; therefore, it is necessary for most women with seizure disorders to continue anticonvulsant therapy during pregnancy. Phenytoin is used by two-thirds of pregnant mothers with treated seizures (Dalessio 1985), but other common anticonvulsants in current use include phenobarbital, primidone (Mysoline), carbamazepine (Tegretol), and ethosuximide (Zarontin). An increased risk of microcephaly, mental retardation, and epilepsy is well documented in the children of epileptic mothers, but it is difficult to distinguish seizure-induced and anticonvulsant-induced intrauterine events.

Trimethadione (Tridione), previously in widespread use for petit mal epilepsy, has been found to produce a syndrome of developmental delay, speech disturbance, and facial anomalies such as low-set ears, irregular teeth, and V-shaped eyebrows (Dalessio 1985; Paulson and Paulson 1981; Zackai et al. 1975). The fetal trimethadione syndrome may also include microcephaly, short stature, and cardiac anomalies.

Phenytoin (Dilantin; formerly diphenylhydantoin) can produce acute neurological side effects (ataxia, nystagmus) and chronic toxicity (gum hyperplasia) in adults and children, but there is also concern

Table 2. Adverse Effects of Anticonvulsants on the Developing Nervous System

Drug	Long-Term Toxic Effects during Pregnancy	Long-Term Toxic Effects during Childhood and Adolescence
trimethadione	developmental delay somatic anomalies	
phenytoin	somatic anomalies ?cerebellar damage ?developmental delay	?cerebellar damage
valproic acid	neural tube defects (spina bifida)	hepatotoxicity
phenobarbital	seemingly harmless	lethargy, mood, cognitive, behavioral disturbance
carbamazepine	seemingly harmless	behavioral stimulation
lithium	cardiovascular and somatic malformations	thyroid dysfunction skin scarring (acne)
alcohol	neurological, behavioral, cognitive, craniofacial, body growth	neurological, behavioral, and hepatic
marijuana	similar to alcohol	?chronic amotivational state

regarding possible neurodevelopmental effects of phenytoin. A fetal hydantoin syndrome has been described, entailing (1) slow body growth, specifically during the intrauterine period; (2) developmental delay; (3) craniofacial anomalies (small nose, depressed nasal bridge, hypertelorism, bowed upper lip); (4) limb anomalies, including hypoplasia of fingers and nails; and (5) other abnormalities, such as cardiac defects and inguinal hernias (Hanson et al. 1976; Hanson and Buehler 1982; Monson et al. 1973). The existence of a specific fetal hydantoin syndrome has been questioned by subsequent studies that have not confirmed a teratogenic link (Dalessio 1985), and by a constellation of similar clinical findings in epileptic women not taking anticonvulsant medication. Seizure-associated fetal hypoxia may be responsible for these changes. The "fetal hydantoin syndrome" may, in fact, be disease-induced rather than drug-induced.

Chronic phenytoin exposure of cultured fetal mouse spinal cord neurons is associated with a diminution in the number of surviving cells (and a dose-dependent decrease in the activity of choline acetyltransferase, the enzyme that synthesizes acetylcholine) (Swaiman et al. 1983), but this in vitro neurotoxicity is not associated with known clinical abnormalities.

Phenobarbital, a sedative-anticonvulsant drug in common use for 60 years, appears to be relatively safe when used during pregnancy, although one study has suggested a slightly increased risk of teratogenicity (Hill and Kleinberg 1984). Mothers using phenobarbital may deliver children with neonatal withdrawal syndrome marked by jitteriness and sleep disturbance, which stops after several days (Desmond et al. 1972). Phenobarbital is used therapeutically in the neonatal period to lower serum bilirubin levels (by inducing hepatic enzymes); long-range consequences of this treatment have not been identified. Similar to phenytoin, chronic phenobarbital exposure of cultured fetal mouse neurons lowers cell survival (Bergey et al. 1981), but no known clinical abnormalities are associated with this demonstrable neurotoxicity. Phenobarbital, whose toxicity in adults and children in acute overdosage can be dangerous and even life-threatening, appears safe in therapeutic range for children and even infants.

Valproic acid (Depakene), available in the United States for nearly a decade, has a recognized potential for serious hepatic toxicity in adults and children. During pregnancy, valproic acid treatment increases the risk of a neural tube defect (American Academy of Pediatrics Committee on Drugs 1983; Dalessio 1985; Jeavons 1984; Tein and MacGregor 1985). The estimated risk for spina bifida is around 1 percent for a woman taking valproic acid during the first trimester of pregnancy. Certain combinations of valproic acid with other drugs may be more teratogenic than valproic acid alone (Jea-vons 1984). The American Academy of Pediatrics Committee on Drugs (1983) recommends that a pregnant woman taking valproic acid consider prenatal testing (measurement of alpha-fetoprotein in blood and/or amniotic fluid) to detect spina bifida or other neural tube defects.

Experimental work with valproic acid in rodents has demonstrated several dose-related teratogenic effects, including kidney abnormal-ities, cleft palate, and encephalocele. In addition, there is a report describing an infant exposed only to valproic acid in utero who had dysmorphic facial features (hypertelorism, prominent forehead, and micrognathia) and growth deficiency (Tein and MacGregor 1985).

For treatment of pregnant women or adolescent girls who may bear children, phenytoin and carbamazepine have been recommended for prevention of grand mal seizures, and ethosuximide for petit mal (Dalessio 1985), with blood samples obtained at regular intervals to ensure therapeutic and subtoxic levels.

In general, intrauterine exposure to anticonvulsants of several dif-ferent chemical categories—or intrauterine seizures—may have long-term adverse effects on a variety of areas of development.

Neuroleptic (antipsychotic) medications, such as phenothiazines, thi-oxanthenes, and butyrophenones, have not been determined to cause morphological teratogenicity in humans (Gelenberg 1984; Nurnberg and Prudic 1984), apart from anecdoctal links that may reflect only chance associations. Long-lasting or permanent effects on behavior in the absence of demonstrable structural changes have been pos-tulated based on animal studies, but demonstrable behavioral tera-togenicity of neuroleptic drugs in humans is not supported by avail-able data (Madsen et al. 1981; Nurnberg and Prudic 1984; Rosengarten and Friedhoff 1979; Vorhees et al. 1979). Intrauterine effects of maternal psychosis have also been postulated, but have not been well documented or compared to risks of early drug treatment.

Lithium, when used during pregnancy, is strongly suspected to cause permanent cardiac abnormalities. Serious lithium-induced tera-togenic effects involve major cardiovascular malformations (Baldes-sarini 1985; Nora et al. 1974; Schou et al. 1973) such as Ebstein's anomaly (malformation of the tricuspid valve, dilatation of the right ventricular outflow tract, and patent ductus arteriosus) as well as rhythmic irregularities, specifically atrial flutter (Wilson et al. 1983). Lithium exposure during the first trimester is associated with a 2 to 3 percent occurrence of Ebstein's anomaly in the offspring (common prevalence is reported as 0.005 percent). Ebstein's anomaly is a major cardiac liability, and leads to death in 95 percent of cases by age 50 years.

Intrauterine exposure to lithium is also associated with a 7 percent risk of all forms of cardiac malformations, and a total prevalence of somatic malformations of 11 percent (compared to 3 to 5 percent in the general population).

Lithium serves as a reminder that psychotropic medications may cause enduring developmental effects on the body outside of the nervous system.

Lithium use by a pregnant mother may also cause some transient effects in the newborn: diabetes insipidus (Morrell et al. 1983) as well as transient hypotonia and hyporeflexia ("floppy baby syndrome") (Morrell et al. 1983; Woody et al. 1971) in the neonate are potential consequences of maternal lithium treatment. Profound hypotonia and depressed deep tendon reflexes were observed until day 6 in an infant who manifested gross motor delays at 1 year (Morrell et al. 1983). These effects of lithium might be linked with an influence on cation exchange across cell membranes, which can cause intracellular hypokalemia and extracellular hyperkalemia (Singer and Rotenberg 1973). These early effects are not known to have an enduring influence in later childhood.

Especially during the first trimester, when cardiac development is critical, discontinuation of lithium is generally advised during pregnancy. However, even in this case of clear teratogenicity, the risk of lithium exposure to the embryo must be measured against potentially life-threatening risks associated with maternal psychosis in certain individuals. Generally, though, other treatment modalities can be employed during pregnancy, such as neuroleptics in low divided doses, electroconvulsive therapy (ECT), or hospitalization.

Diazepam (Valium) use during early pregnancy appeared linked with cleft lip and cleft palate in initial studies. More recently, a case-control study (Rosenberg et al. 1980) and a prospective study involving 33,249 pregnant women and their offspring (Shiono and Mills 1984) found no association between diazepam and oral clefts.

There are a wide variety of other teratogenic agents, but one of particular prominence regarding neurotoxic effects is isotretinoin.

Isotretinoin (Accutane), a retinoic acid analog of vitamin A used for treating severe cystic acne, can cause major malformations of the central nervous system (Lammer et al. 1985). First-trimester exposure is associated with hydrocephalus, holoprosencephaly, microcephaly, cerebellar hypoplasia, and morphogenic errors of cortical and cerebellar neuronal migration. Craniofacial anomalies (most commonly microtia or anotia) and cardiac defects (such as transposition of the great vessels and tetralogy of Fallot) are also described. Studies in mice suggest that retinoic acid exerts toxic influences on cephalic neural-crest cells similar to those attributed to alcohol and thalidomide.

In summary, the intrauterine period—particularly the first trimester—appears to be a time of maximal vulnerability of the central nervous system for permanent structural defects resulting from toxic exposures. A large variety of medications and agents can exert developmental neurotoxic influences during embryonic and fetal life, including thalidomide, tetracycline, alcohol, marijuana, anticonvulsants, lithium, and isotretinoin.

There is no currently known teratogenic risk concerning antidepressants, neuroleptics, psychostimulants, barbiturates, or benzodiazepines in general.

Inhibition of protein synthesis and calcium channel blockade are implicated as possible teratogenic mediators for some agents, but the teratogenic mechanisms remain to be clarified for most toxins.

The experience with thalidomide and isotretinoin underscores the risk of drugs used in women of childbearing age, particularly during adolescence when unplanned or impulsive pregnancy is a high risk.

Even in a brief review of teratology, it is clear that careful empirical research is needed to distinguish drug-induced and disease-induced phenomena. Some so-called drug-induced effects may be instead due to the underlying disease, and some drug effects may be less dangerous than disease effects.

The intrauterine period, a time of extreme developmental vulnerability of the brain and other organs, requires special attention to prevent enduring anatomical effects of early exposure to medications and toxins.

BIRTH

The consequences of anesthesia and analgesia during labor and delivery have been questioned for over 100 years. Drugs used routinely during labor and delivery can generally affect the behavior of newborns in a dose-related and transient manner (Golub and Golub 1981). Studies investigating the influence of obstetric medications have been typically designed to observe effects within the first week or, occasionally, consequences 1 month or more after delivery.

Phenobarbital, a drug no longer used routinely for obstetric purposes, depresses respiratory centers of the brain and may delay the newborn's initiation of breathing; it also can cause lethargy for several days (Scanlon and Hollenbeck 1983). Naloxone, an opiate antagonist, administered just before delivery, is effective in preventing perinatal respiratory and behavioral depression caused by the commonly used analgesic meperidine. There appear to be no long-lasting direct pharmacological effects of these agents, although large-scale prospective studies have not been reported.

It is not only the baby's behavior that can be influenced by obstetric drugs, but parent-child interactions can be altered as well. A sedated or irritable newborn may evoke different parental patterns of stimulation and interaction. As the mother's perinatal sedative or analgesic medication dosage increases, the baby's activity may diminish; in response, the mother's activity is found to increase, and the father's activity decreases (Scanlon and Hollenbeck 1983). Speculatively, obstetric medication may influence the parents' initial impressions of the child and exert a developmental influence that, in some cases, may have long-term implications for the child's future behavior.

In a review of studies of long-term effects of obstetric medication, Scanlon and Hollenbeck (1983) did not find evidence of significant consequences. In a study of babies delivered by emergency cesarean section under general anesthesia, compared to babies delivered vaginally without general anesthesia, behavioral differences observed at 8 months did not seem due to a medication effect, but instead were attributed to the obstetric circumstances necessitating cesarean section and the mother's experience of an emergency operative delivery (Field and Widmayer 1980).

It is possible that a drug interaction between diphenhydramine (Benadryl) and temazepam (Restoril) may lead to an increased infant mortality just prior to delivery (Kargas et al. 1985). This newly reported perinatal drug effect has not been confirmed, but it underscores that physiological events at parturition may entail specific time-limited pharmacological vulnerabilities. (See further discussion in Chapter 3.)

Enduring pharmacologic effects of obstetric and perinatally administered drugs have been hypothesized, but not definitively demonstrated (Kraemer et al. 1985). However, medications administered during labor and delivery may alter the human experience and behavior around birth, which may have a lasting emotional influence for certain individuals.

INFANCY AND EARLY CHILDHOOD

In contrast to the considerable teratogenic risk many drugs pose for the fetus, the period of infancy and early childhood presents fewer structural risks but many long-term behavioral and cognitive risks. During this period, children are exposed to many medications, commonly used for treatment of various medical disorders of infancy and early childhood. Yet, the vulnerability of the developing brain is dramatically lessened after birth.

Phenobarbital is widely used in pediatrics for preventing febrile seizures. Approximately 5 percent of children between 6 months and 5 years of age experience brief (less than 15 minutes) generalized convulsions within 24 hours of the onset of fever. Most children will outgrow their febrile seizures, but some children are placed on anticonvulsant prophylaxis because of complicating features such as frequent or prolonged febrile seizures, coexisting focal seizures, developmental delays, or neurological abnormalities. Most children treated for febrile seizures are placed on phenobarbital maintenance for 1 to 4 years.

Two major concerns have surfaced with the use of phenobarbital in infancy and early childhood: (1) development of behavior disorders, primarily hyperkinetic and attentional syndromes, and (2) adverse effects on cognition, due to sedation or direct attentional interference (Reynolds 1983; Schmidt 1984).

The appearance of impulsivity or behavior disturbance in children using phenobarbital is not a clear-cut or established phenomenon. Of 109 children treated with phenobarbital following a first febrile seizure, 42 percent developed a behavioral disorder, usually a hyperkinetic syndrome, whereas 18 percent of children with febrile seizures who were not placed on phenobarbital developed behavior disorders (Wolf and Forsythe 1978). In another study, 3 of 35 children on phenobarbital had side effects of daytime fussiness and sleep disruption (awakening several hours early in the morning), but did not show hyperactivity (Camfield et al. 1979). By contrast, younger children (less than 2 years old) who were hospitalized with a first febrile seizure showed behavioral disturbances after 3 to 9 weeks whether placed on phenobarbital, phenytoin, or placebo; these behavioral effects were interpreted as due to hospitalization and illness (Bacon et al. 1981). Phenobarbital may increase the impulsivity or behavior problems of some children, but careful evaluation of the individual child would be needed to document other clinically confounding factors.

Cognitive effects of phenobarbital have also been difficult to identify (Reynolds 1983; Trimble 1981). Early in the course of treatment (first several days), sedation may interfere with attentiveness and learning. During chronic treatment, toxic blood levels of phenobarbital may be present intermittently during periods of dehydration or persistently as commonly occurs when valproic acid is added to a regimen with phenobarbital. On a long-term basis, such persistent unrecognized elevations can be associated with cognitive impairment and have adverse developmental consequences ("pseudo-retardation"). Even in the therapeutic range, some cognitive price may be paid. In young children (ages 2 to 5 years) assessed with the Bayley Scales of Infant Development and the Stanford-Binet Intelligence Scale, detrimental effects of phenobarbital in the therapeutic range were found on memory (related to serum concentration of drug) and comprehension (linked with duration of therapy) (Camfield et al. 1979). However, the validity of this study has been challenged (Fishman 1979).

Phenobarbital treatment in infancy might contribute to development of long-term behavior problems, inattention, or impulsivity— but these developmental effects may represent consequences of disease-associated neurodevelopmental disabilities. Alternatively, certain of these effects may be due to other associated processes, such as hospitalization or emotional upset. Long-term use of acutely cognition-reducing or impulsivity-generating drugs may lead to serious impairments in learning and behavior, but there is no evidence of direct developmental neurotoxicity produced by phenobarbital after 60 years of clinical use.

Valproic acid, in addition to its teratogenic effects on neural tube formation, has an unusual but significant hepatotoxicity. Used in treatment of absence and other types of seizures, valproic acid may cause the idiosyncratic formation of hepatotoxic metabolites, which can lead to acute hepatic failure and, potentially, death. This metabolic reaction is uncommon, is not due to immunological hypersensitivity, is not dose-dependent (may be seen at low doses), appears more likely when valproic acid is used in combination with other drugs, and may be due to mitochondrial enzyme inhibition (Gram and Bentsen 1985; Powell-Jackson et al. 1984; Rimmer and Richens 1985).

Fetal hepatotoxicity of valproic acid has been described mainly in children, with 75 percent of reported cases below age 10 years (Rothner 1985; Zafrani and Berthelot 1982; Zimmerman and Ishak 1982), but this pattern may reflect the typical age of valproic acid use. However, using commercial marketing estimates to correct for age of use, the main vulnerability appears greater in young children under age 2 years on multiple drug therapy (risk 1/500), whereas there is a low risk (1/45,000) for individuals above age 2 years using valproic acid alone (Dreifuss 1987). Many children under age 2 years who receive valproic acid in combination with other anticonvulsants have major developmental and neurological abnormalities, had failed on single anticonvulsant treatments, and may be viewed as comprising a high-risk medical group (Dreifuss et al. 1987).

The hepatotoxicity is usually seen during the first half-year of treatment, so it is recommended that liver function tests (including blood ammonia), hematological indices, and clinical status (seizures, headache, lassitude, abdominal discomfort, vomiting, facial edema, and jaundice) receive close surveillance for the first 6 months of valproic acid therapy.

Valproic acid is a simple branched-chain fatty acid, a novel agent that differs in chemical structure from any other commercially available drug. Valproate-induced hepatotoxicity may be due to a rare genetic or defective enzymatic reaction in fatty acid metabolism (Mortensen 1980; Thurston and Hauhart 1987; Zimmerman and Ishak 1982).

In view of the putative age-related vulnerability, the current data may serve as a warning that new drugs involving fatty acid metabolism may need to be monitored for special risk in children.

Phenytoin has been the focus of a debate regarding cerebellar atrophy. The acute motor incoordination of phenytoin intoxication suggests that the cerebellum is a target site of phenytoin action. Cerebellar Purkinje cell loss has been cited as evidence of an adverse effect of phenytoin on the cerebellum, but such cell loss antedates the use of phenytoin (Schmidt 1984). Alternatively, seizure-induced hypoxia may be responsible, but computed tomography (CT) scans of adults treated with phenytoin for seizures (compared to persons scanned because of headache) failed to show cerebellar atrophy attributable to epilepsy or drug (Ballenger et al. 1982).

Atrophy of the cerebellum did, however, appear after phenytoin intoxication in a man without seizures who was treated prophylactically after a subarachnoid hemorrhage (Lindvall and Nilsson 1984). CT scans before and after a several-month period of phenytoin toxicity demonstrated development of marked cerebellar atrophy. Clinical signs of cerebellar dysfunction were initially severe, but still persisted (although to a lesser degree) 6 years after phenytoin intoxication, and 5 years after cessation of anticonvulsant treatment. In a study of 7 children, long-term use of phenytoin with high blood levels (exceeding 30 mg/liter in at least 4 at times) was implicated as causing permanent ataxia correlated with CT scan evidence of cerebellar atrophy, particularly in the region of the vermis (Baier et al. 1984).

From a practical standpoint, the development of clinical signs of cerebellar dysfunction or radiographic evidence of cerebellar atrophy (CT or nuclear magnetic resonance imaging), even with phenytoin blood levels in the therapeutic range, should lead to consideration of change to another drug.

This ongoing debate can serve to remind us that the apparent effects of a drug may represent signs either of the underlying disease or of covert drug toxicity—and that careful empirical studies are required to determine true clinical effects.

Hexachlorophene is a widely used antibacterial agent, which, after several decades, was found to be highly neurotoxic. Absorption through damaged skin (e.g., cuts, burns, eczema) is possible at all ages, but hexachlorophene constitutes a special risk for young children because of its use in routine daily care. Infants have been exposed to topical hexachlorophene through whole-body bathing, hexachlorophene-containing diaper powders (for treatment of excoriated rash), and in the treatment of burns. Premature infants have been found to absorb hexachlorophene more readily through intact skin than older children. Oral intake of hexachlorophene is unusual, but occurs in the treatment of some intestinal parasites and through accidental overdose, with potentially fatal outcome (Herskowitz and Rosman 1979; Lustig 1963). Neurological symptoms include extreme irritability, seizures, diminished responsiveness to painful stimulation, paralysis, and decreased level of consciousness that may progress to coma or death. Autopsy studies have demonstrated a toxic effect on myelin in the central nervous system (Towfighi 1980), producing edema manifested by vacuolation of white matter.

Hexachlorophene is no longer available in high concentration for antibacterial use in the United States. Teratogenicity of hexachlorophene in humans (including the effects of chronic low level exposure, as for operating room personnel) has not been definitely established. Avoidance of its use during pregnancy is advised (Hill and Kleinberg 1984).

Hexachlorophene provides an example of neurotoxicity occurring without expectation with a seemingly innocuous agent, and whose risk is present at all ages. It is particularly a risk for premature and very young infants due to their increased absorption of topical hexachlorophene. However, after accounting for different levels of exposure, it is not established that there is an increased neurotoxic risk in developing children. The dangers of this drug were not anticipated from the animal literature, and its risk for brain development was not inferred from its primary use or previously known pharmacology.

LATER CHILDHOOD

By age 2 to 3 years, the rate of brain growth has slowed considerably. More than half of the growth toward an adult head circumference is achieved by the end of the first year. Yet, brain growth progresses until around 18 years, and myelination continues through at least the third decade. There is a continuing vulnerability of the developing nervous system in the period of later childhood and adolescence, and first exposures to some chemical agents may occur during this time.

Food colorings, artificial flavors, preservatives, and natural salicylates have elicited much concern because of their widespread occurrence as food additives in the diets of children, particularly in Western countries, and their possible role in altering behavior. Feingold (1974) proposed that one-half or more of children considered hyperactive would benefit from dietary measures that eliminate artificial coloring agents, synthetic food dyes, and certain fruits and vegetables (e.g., apples, oranges, and tomatoes) containing salicylates.

Controlled studies have yielded several findings. Minimal or equivocal results have been found in most children in large-scale studies (Harley et al. 1978a, 1978b). No effects of the Feingold diet have been demonstrated even in cases where mothers' prior observations suggested it would be effective (Mattes and Gittelman-Klein 1978). A small number of hyperactive or attentionally disordered children have been identified with adverse behavioral or learning responses to challenges with artificial food dyes (Swanson and Kinsbourne 1980; Weiss et al. 1980). The clinical characteristics and dose sensitivity of this subgroup remain to be defined.

A biochemical basis for these putative effects has not been determined, but Red Dye No. 3 has been shown to interfere with the uptake of monoaminergic neurotransmitters in synaptosomal preparations (Lafferman and Silbergeld 1979). It is unclear whether apparently dye-sensitive hyperkinetic children are behaviorally or biochemically distinct from other behavior-disordered children, but there might be a subgroup of such children in whom the acute behavioral effects of dietary agents may exert a chronic behavioral-developmental influence.

The clinical relevance of dye consumption for the majority of these children is undetermined. There are no data documenting any behavioral effects of dietary salicylates.

Lead is another environmental agent with potential for neurotoxicity, particularly in children. The neurological consequences of acute lead encephalopathy, seen clinically in children who have ingested lead-containing house paints, are profound: seizures, mental retardation, hemiparesis, coma (associated with increased intracranial pressure), and death. As screening programs to measure blood lead concentration have become established widely in the United States, lead encephalopathy has become a rarity. Lead is still present in some gasolines and in paint of older homes, and low-level chronic toxicity may be seen in children who are apparently asymptomatic (Needleman et al. 1979; Ernhart et al. 1981).

To define the effect of "subclinical" levels of lead, Needleman et al. (1979) compared 58 children with elevated tooth lead levels and 100 children with low-lead levels. Full-scale IQ scores of the high-lead children were lower by 4.5 points (mean scores: 102.1 versus 106.6). In classroom behavior, teachers reported that high-lead children manifested symptoms of attention deficit-hyperactivity disorder: distractibility, impersistence, disorganization, hyperactivity, impulsivity, easy frustration, daydreaming, and difficulty in following directions. Rutter (1980) accepted the findings of cognitive impairment, but not the evidence for behavioral change. An independent panel (Expert Committee on Pediatric Neurobehavioral Evaluations 1983) concluded that current investigations were inconclusive regarding both the neuropsychological deficits and behavioral abnormalities resulting from low-level lead exposure in children.

Since lead may injure endothelial cells and raise intracranial pressure (Krigman et al. 1980; Winder and Kitchen 1984), screening programs remain valuable to prevent the catastrophic consequences of acute lead encephalopathy and to maintain public awareness of lead as a potentially damaging neurotoxin.

Anticonvulsant drugs have possible teratogenic effects as noted above, but may also exert a long-term behavioral effect during childhood.

Phenobarbital can produce a syndrome of excitement, irritability, tearfulness, or aggressive behavior at any age (Stores 1975). These are acute and reversible effects seen in adults and children. However, used in long-term therapy, these acute effects may induce progressive and cumulative effects on behavior and cognition in school-age children.

Carbamazepine has also been associated with adverse behavioral reactions in children. After 4 days to several weeks of treatment, behavioral changes included extreme irritability, agitation, insomnia, and aggressive outbursts in 7 of 200 children (6 to 18 years old) (Silverstein et al. 1982). The tricyclic structure of carbamazepine might contribute to the behavioral toxicity observed because the changes are similar to a behavioral activation (similar to manic switch), which may occur with antidepressant medication; gradual reintroduction of carbamazepine was possible, however, without return of the previously encountered adverse behavioral reactions in 5 of 7 children. No clear developmental effects of carbamazepine are described, apart from known side effects seen in adults.

Methylphenidate or d-*amphetamine* are used in 2 to 3 percent of the American public school population for treatment of attention deficit-hyperactivity disorder. Among several controversial aspects of this treatment, there is concern regarding interference with growth in height and weight. Safer et al. (1972) initially described 29 hyperactive children, taking d-amphetamine or methylphenidate, who showed a decrease in average weight gain. Among 5 of 9 children taking medication for at least 2 years, this reduction in weight gain was accompanied by a decrease in height gain, although to a lesser degree. When medication was discontinued for the summer, a gain in weight was observed, with a "rebound" over expected averages. On the other hand, Gross (1976) found no stunting of growth in 100 children treated for an average of 5 years with methylphenidate, d-amphetamine, or tricyclic antidepressant agents (an alternative treatment for attention deficit-hyperactivity disorder). Mattes and Gittelman (1983) found significant and progressive diminution of height gain among 86 severely disruptive, hyperactive prepubertal children who received methylphenidate (average daily dosage 40 to 50 mg) for up to 4 years. Medication was discontinued in many instances during the summer. Height percentiles dropped from the first through the fourth years of therapy: 1.4 percentile points after the first year (not significant), 8.1 percentile points after the second year, 13 points after the third, and 18 after the fourth. For example, a boy at the 50th percentile at the beginning of the study would be at the 32nd percentile after 4 years of methylphenidate treatment, a loss of 1.3 inches (3.3 cm) anticipated if the child had remained at the 50th percentile. In general, 1 to 3 cm of height and 1 to 3 kg of weight maximally are not gained over several years of treatment. Overall, suppression of linear growth was proportional to dosage and to the child's initial height, so that taller children "lost" more height. Less than 2 percent of the variance in adult height can be attributed to psychostimulant treatment (Mattes and Gittelman 1983). It is unclear whether drug holidays help, or whether any one medication is preferred.

Neuroendocrine studies of hyperactive children treated with stimulants assessing growth hormone, prolactin, and somatomedin have not yet elucidated a hormonal basis for changes in growth rate (Schultz et al. 1982; Shaywitz et al. 1982).

Despite conflicting results in these population studies of children, growth effects may be significant for individual children receiving stimulant therapy. It is clinically sensible to plot weight and height regularly (at least two or three times yearly) using standard growth curves for children, looking for a decrease in height percentile during stimulant therapy. Slowing of weight gain is typically transient and rarely a clinical problem, but a persistent height effect would require management based on the individual's situation. Reducing dosage, providing longer drug holidays, switching to another drug, or discontinuing medication may be considered.

Unlike the long series of drugs discussed so far, the effect of psychostimulants on growth cannot be attributed to the underlying disease and is not merely a cumulative effect of long-term use of an acutely sedating drug. This effect might, or might not, be the result of its neuropharmacological properties. Although the mechanism is still unclear, the magnitude of this drug-induced effect appears generally small. Most clinicians would consider this growth effect to be an acceptable disadvantage for children whose attention deficit-hyperactivity disorder may be a serious problem in their development. Nonetheless, the influence of psychostimulants on body growth, although still being documented, is one of the important developmental pharmacotoxic effects in medicine.

Aspirin, with its apparent association with Reye's syndrome, provides another important illustration of a drug with toxic effects in childhood not generally seen in adulthood (Hurwitz et al. 1985). Reye's syndrome is defined as (1) an acute noninflammatory encephalopathy characterized by an altered level of consciousness, generally lethargy or coma, in the absence of cerebrospinal fluid (CSF) leukocytosis and (2) liver involvement, as documented by fatty changes on microscopic examination or at least a threefold elevation in serum liver function tests (SGOT, SGPT, or ammonia) (Rogers et al. 1985). In 1984, 190 new cases in the United States were reported to the Centers for Disease Control (1985), and 85 percent were below age 15 (29 percent, 0 to 4 years; 18 percent, 5 to 9 years; 38 percent, 10 to 14 years).

Although prospective studies have not been completed, retrospective case-control studies have strongly associated Reye's syndrome with aspirin use during the 2-week prodromal phase, often for treatment of influenza or varicella infection (American Academy of Pediatrics Committee on Infectious Diseases 1982; Rogers et al. 1985; Starko et al. 1980). Medical recommendations for curtailing aspirin use in childhood appear to have contributed to a drop in the reported number of new cases of Reye's syndrome (American Academy of Pediatrics Committee on Infectious Diseases 1982; Rogers et al. 1985).

The reason for the special sensitivity of children is unknown, but this is a major example—along with psychostimulants and perhaps valproic acid and hexachlorophene—of a developmental pharmacotoxic effect.

Tricyclic antidepressants have been commonly used by pediatricians for treatment of enuresis in children, and are now becoming increasingly used in higher doses for treatment of affective and other disorders in children. Since tricyclic antidepressants share some pharmacological properties with psychostimulants (particularly regarding facilitation of catecholamine neurotransmission), there is a hypothetical possibility that growth suppression might be produced by antidepressant treatments in children.

Since treatment of major depression is typically only several months in duration, there is presumably ample opportunity for continuing growth after completion of drug therapy. Antidepressant treatment of childhood depression would, therefore, present a smaller risk of enduring growth effects than psychostimulant treatment of attention deficit-hyperactivity disorder, which commonly is several years in duration.

For the depressed children and adolescents whose antidepressant treatment may need to be maintained for more than a year, the theoretical potential (not empirically demonstrated) of drug effects on height and weight might need consideration in treatment decisions.

Antidepressant treatments in children may be associated with an increase in dental caries. The anticholinergic properties of these drugs may interfere with salivation, and produce a subjective sense of "dry mouth" (xerostomia). If dental hygiene is not adequate, the reduced salivary flow may lead to increased plaque accumulation and formation of cavities. Especially for children who have not yet acquired healthy habits of dental hygiene, this may pose a significant problem. If antidepressant treatment induces "dry mouth," an agent with relatively less anticholinergic properties (such as desipramine or nortriptyline) can be tried, and provisions for careful dental care should be assured. Sugar-free gum or candy may be helpful in stimulating saliva flow. Daily brushings with fluoride toothpaste, flossing, and routine dental care visits are generally adequate to deal with this problem. Drug-induced xerostomia in association with insufficient dental hygiene may produce enduring dental symptomatology.

Neuroleptic (antipsychotic) drugs are in widespread and generally cautious use in children, but some children have developed withdrawal-emergent dyskinesia and fewer have developed persistent tardive dyskinesia. Despite concern about long-term developmental effects of these dyskinesias, none have been demonstrated. Neuroleptic-associated dyskinesia, presumably associated with supersensitivity of dopamine receptors particularly in the basal ganglia, is manifested by involuntary choreoathetoid movements that typically affect the face and limbs, including orofacial dyskinesia, chorea, athetosis, dystonia, facial grimacing, blepharospasm, and tic-like movements (Jeste and Wyatt 1982). Neuroleptic-associated dyskinesia, defined by development of the movement disorder after at least 3 months' cumulative neuroleptic exposure, is subtyped according to time course: (1) withdrawal emergent (associated with decrease in neuroleptic dosage), (2) transient (resolving within 3 months without reinstitution of medication or dosage increase), and (3) persistent (longer than 3 months) (Schooler and Kane 1982). All three forms of dyskinesia can occur in children and adolescents (Gualtieri et al. 1980, 1984; Polizos et al. 1973; Tarsy and Baldessarini 1984, 1986). No particular antipsychotic agent is proven to present less risk for developing these dyskinesias, although high doses of potent agents may be especially risky (Baldessarini et al. 1987).

Tardive dyskinesia has been documented in adolescents and children after only 5 months of therapy (Caine et al. 1978; Gualtieri et al. 1980; Jeste and Wyatt 1982; Polizos et al. 1973; Tarsy and Baldessarini 1984, 1986). The prevalence of tardive dyskinesia among children and adolescents on long-term neuroleptic treatment in several studies is 8 to 20 percent (Jeste and Wyatt 1982). The effects of dosage and duration of neuroleptic therapy in children (as well as adults) are still being defined (Gualtieri et al. 1984; Tarsy and Baldessarini 1986).

Polizos et al. (1973) studied the clinical effects of withdrawing neuroleptic drugs in institutionalized psychotic children, ages 6 to 12 years, who had been treated for 6 to 15 months with drugs such as fluphenazine (mean treatment length, 14 months; mean daily dosage, 25 mg) and thioridazine (13 months, 400 mg). A withdrawal-emergent syndrome of involuntary movements and ataxia was seen in 14 of 34 children, with onset at 1 to 15 days after drug discontinuation. The neurological symptoms remitted spontaneously in half the children, and for the others within 2 weeks of restarting neuroleptic medication.

In their study of 41 children, adolescents, and young adults (mostly mentally retarded), Gualtieri et al. (1984) found that 44 percent had neuroleptic-associated neurobehavioral problems: tardive dyskinesia, withdrawal dyskinesia, nondyskinetic withdrawal symptoms, or transient behavioral deterioration. Of the three cases of tardive dyskinesia, two remitted spontaneously within 9 months; one persisted after 12 months of follow-up. The other neuroleptic-induced adverse effects resolved in the other 38 patients within 8 weeks. Only 12 of the 41 required resumption of neuroleptics. In these data, the risk of persistent tardive dyskinesia was 2.5 percent; the majority of these individuals did not need continuing neuroleptic treatment.

Discontinuation of antipsychotic medication is the only known effective treatment for tardive dyskinesia, although clinical situations may justify continued use in some individuals. In general, neuroleptic medication should be used only when clinically essential. Doses should be as low as possible, with reevaluation every 3 to 6 months regarding continuing need for medication (American Psychiatric Association Task Force on Late Neurological Effects of Antipsychotic Drugs 1980). Drug-free "neuroleptic holidays" may lessen the risk of developing tardive dyskinesia (Gualtieri and Guimond 1981), but intermittent therapy has not been evaluated in children or adults, and could conceivably be harmful.

A possible behavioral counterpart to tardive dyskinesia has been observed in children, adolescents, and young adults. Psychosis, elation, euphoria, and hyperactivity have been reported following discontinuation of neuroleptic medication (Gualtieri and Guimond 1981). Supersensitivity of dopamine receptors in the mesolimbic system has been speculated to underlie these behavioral and emotional changes (Schooler and Kane 1982). It is conceivable that more subtle cognitive and affective phenomena may emerge in a "tardive" manner during chronic neuroleptic treatment. Such changes would need to be clinically distinguished from the disease-related effects associated with the natural course of illness.

Although the documented risks of tardive dyskinesia may appear lower in children than adults, this may be the result of lower dosages, shorter durations of treatment, or more cautious monitoring in children; these parameters have not yet been decisively examined.

At this time, there is no definitive evidence that children are at greater or lesser risk for withdrawal-emergent or tardive dyskinesia than adults, after accounting for their different levels of exposure (i.e., dosage and duration of treatment). Despite the reportedly greater short-term risk of dystonic and parkinsonian extrapyramidal reactions in adolescents (Keepers et al. 1983; see also Chapter 3), a long-term age-specific pharmacotoxicity of neuroleptic agents in children has not been described.

Dental hygiene should be emphasized for children receiving neuroleptics because the anticholinergic properties may promote caries formation. Given the lengthy treatments with neuroleptics that some children receive, dental care as well as neurological observation should be emphasized as a routine part of ongoing treatment.

Generally, the period of childhood does not present the same degree of gross vulnerability to structural change seen during the intrauterine period. The increased sensitivity of children to aspirin (hepatotoxicity of Reye's syndrome) and possibly hexachlorophene (neurotoxic effects on myelin) and valproic acid (hepatotoxicity) points to an age-related vulnerability and to the value of epidemiological studies in the evaluation of therapeutic and toxic effects of drugs. Anticholinergic side effects of antidepressants and neuroleptics on the formation of dental cavities should be monitored, and careful dental hygiene is recommended. The effects of psychostimulants on weight and height in some children represent a specifically developmental problem, namely growth suppression. With this category of drugs, the risk of adverse effects must be measured against the potential developmental benefit for the individual.

ADOLESCENCE

Many of the same issues discussed regarding school-age children pertain to adolescents as well, but the hepatotoxicity of aspirin and valproic acid are probably seen at lower rates. There are also some additional considerations that apply in adolescence.

Psychostimulants may continue to suppress physical growth in the adolescent period. This effect is reversible on cessation of drug therapy during childhood and early adolescence. However, with epiphyseal closing of the long bones at ages 17 to 21, psychostimulants in late adolescence may cause permanent stunting of height due to a lack of opportunity for posttreatment growth. Psychostimulants (and speculatively antidepressants) may be used with attentive risk-benefit evaluation during the period of epiphyseal closing, when there may be a generally small but permanent effect on body height.

Lithium has an increasing role in the pediatric psychopharmacological armamentarium, particularly among adolescents with bipolar disorder and aggressive behavior, as well as among some younger children with severe temper tantrums (Davis 1979; DeLong 1978; Rapoport et al. 1978). The nervous system is involved in some short-term adverse effects of lithium, such as tremor, blurred vision, weakness, confusion, "spaceyness," and "forgetting." Acute intoxication may occur at blood levels not far above therapeutic range and is characterized by vomiting, dysarthria, ataxia, coma, and seizures (Baldessarini 1984, 1985). Moreover, severe acute intoxication can be associated with sustained brain and kidney damage.

Lithium treatment in adults may lead to transient kidney dysfunction (polyuria or diabetes insipidus), which is usually clinically mild, modifiable by diuretics, and reversible on cessation of treatment. Initial reports of major renal functional impairment resulting from chronic lithium treatment were not confirmed by more controlled prospective studies (Amsterdam et al. 1985; Bendz 1985; Imbs et al. 1986; Johnson et al. 1984; Smigan et al. 1984; Vestergaard and Amdisen 1981), and the changes now appear less severe than effects of nonsteroidal anti-inflammatory drugs (e.g., aspirin). There is some demonstrable structural injury, but the histological changes are generally mild. The risk and significance of these findings are now believed to be minor (American Psychiatric Association Task Force on Long-term Effects of Lithium on the Kidney 1987). Some instances of long-term renal effects observed in lithium-treated adults may be due to their undertreatment of concurrent medical illnesses, such as hypertension, diabetes, kidney infection or obstruction, and analgesic abuse (Heninger 1984). The possibility of chronic renal effects in children must be considered, and careful monitoring of kidney function before and during lithium therapy (minimally, blood creatinine every 3 months) is advised (Popper 1985).

In addition, extended use of lithium in adults can result in goiter and occasionally clinical hypothyroidism (Lindstedt et al. 1977; Perrild et al. 1984). Presumably, children would be similarly vulnerable to the intrinsic antithyroid properties of lithium, which would be potentially more significant and hazardous in growing children than adults. Careful initial evaluation—baseline levels of thyroxine, T3 uptake, and thyroid stimulating hormone (TSH)—and periodic thyroid assessments—TSH every 4 months, full battery every year—are recommended (Popper 1985). Prompt reevaluation of thyroid function would be suggested in case of emerging clinical evidence of hypothyroidism, such as lassitude, unexplained weight gain, decline in school performance, or inattention.

Long-term lithium therapy may also be associated with a shift in calcium metabolism, marked by calcium mobilization from bones (Jefferson et al. 1987). Although this is rarely a clinical problem in adults, it theoretically might be more of a problem in children. Sensible observation might include periodic measurements of height (bone growth) as well as calcium, phosphorus, and alkaline phosphatase levels, which would permit a metabolic correction.

During adolescence, acne is a common problem influencing skin, self-image, and self-esteem. Among several skin problems induced by lithium, aggravation of acne is a potential complication of lithium therapy in adolescents. Lithium may worsen the clinical course of the acne or reduce the effectiveness of acne treatment. For routine acne occurring during lithium therapy, standard skin treatments are generally sufficient. For the unusual cases whose severity suggests a risk of scarring, lithium should be used cautiously, and acne should be treated aggressively to avoid permanent skin damage. Isotretinoin

(Accutane) may be an effective adjunct to lithium therapy when the acne is severe, but its teratogenic properties require caution for adolescent girls who may become pregnant. In extreme cases, inadequate management of lithium-induced acne may lead to permanent physical sequelae.

The possibility of permanent neurological deficit due to lithium has been raised. There are case reports of adults receiving lithium, without other psychotropic agents, who manifested persistent motor symptoms and memory disturbances following severe lithium intoxication (Apte and Langston 1983; Hartitzsch et al. 1972).

The cognitive effects of lithium in childhood and adolescence have undergone limited investigation. Platt et al. (1984) studied 61 children between 5 and 13 years of age and found that lithium did not have pronounced adverse effects on cognition except in five children (8 percent) who showed a significant decrement in performance on the Porteus Maze Test. The characteristics of this subgroup were not further defined. Overall, lithium had significantly fewer cognitive adverse effects than haloperidol and was recommended for consideration in children with conduct disorders characterized by extreme aggressiveness for whom nonpharmacological therapies are ineffective.

Some aspects of lithium toxicity may depend on use of concurrent medication. In patients who are receiving lithium and antipsychotic agents, the antiemetic actions of neuroleptics might blunt nausea and vomiting that occur in moderately severe lithium intoxication (Baldessarini 1984, 1985). Also, iodine-containing compounds, such as cough medicines or bronchodilators, may be problematic by increasing the risk of goiter.

Lithium blood levels are highly sensitive to variations in dietary intake of salt. Several days of low salt intake can push therapeutic blood levels into a toxic range, or large salt ingestions can cause a drop in lithium blood levels and a return of behavioral symptoms ("taco tantrums"). Certain adolescents and children have an erratic consumption of "junk foods" or large variations in exercise; therefore, diet- and exertion-induced shifts in salt and fluid balance should be anticipated, and these patients should be followed carefully for untoward rises or falls in their blood levels during lithium therapy.

Lithium presents some technical challenges for effective dosing of adolescents and children. The effects are generally transient, although lithium toxicity can present acute risk. At present, lithium appears to have limited long-term effects on kidney function, although this question may be considered unsettled. In contrast, there is definite reason for concern regarding lithium-aggravated acne and caries, which may have enduring effects in certain cases. Such dangers, however, can be generally avoided by standard medical care.

Adolescence completes the cycle, since pregnancy, planned or otherwise, carries risks of toxic exposures to recreational drugs (alcohol and marijuana), isotretinoin (treatment of acne), and other agents.

SUMMARY

A developmental framework is critical for understanding neurotoxicological risks. Prior to conception, exposure to certain drugs or toxins can have a cytotoxic effect, which may present as abortion or infertility rather than developmental disorder.

After conception, the intrauterine period is a time of extreme neurodevelopmental vulnerability, requiring special care to prevent enduring anatomical effects. Tetracycline and thalidomide are examples that show that teratological risk cannot always be inferred from animal studies or experience with adults. Lithium and certain anticonvulsant drugs present clear or strongly suspected dangers to prenatal development. Given the present level of clinical and epidemiological knowledge, neuroleptics, antidepressants, psychostimulants, and minor tranquilizers generally appear to be safe during pregnancy. Drug interactions (e.g., alcohol and marijuana) may be critical in the appearance of teratological effects, and the biochemical events may interact with environmental and social influences such as malnutrition and poverty (access to medical care) in the expression of neurotoxicological symptomatology.

At birth, drugs used in obstetrics do not appear to have enduring neurotoxic or somatic effects. However, medications administered during labor and delivery may alter the infant's behavior and the parents' response to the infant, and could have a lasting emotional impact in certain individuals.

In contrast to the extreme vulnerability during embryonic and fetal life, the period of early childhood poses much fewer structural risks to the child's growing body and brain, but there are long-term behavioral and cognitive risks. During this period, children are exposed to many medications for treatment of the various medical disorders of infancy and early childhood. The long-term use of acutely sedating drugs may have progressive and cumulative effects on arousal, behavior, and learning. Several anticonvulsants may have neurotoxic effects, and toxic influences on the liver and other organs. Valproic acid will require special attention because this recently introduced drug was quickly found to have a major hepatotoxicity; this drug may present a higher risk for children, who may have a greater likelihood of idiosyncratic defects in fatty acid metabolism. A similar mechanism may be involved in the potentially severe hepatotoxicity of Reye's syndrome, which may follow use of aspirin. The antibacterial agent hexachlorophene provides an example of a seemingly innocuous agent with considerable neurotoxicity, whose dangers for brain development were not inferred from its primary use or its previously known pharmacology, and whose risk may be greater for premature and young infants than for children and adults.

In later childhood, food colorings appear to be generally safe, but might adversely influence behavior or learning in a susceptible subgroup. Lead is a known neurotoxin, and perhaps can also influence behavior and learning even below overtly neurotoxic levels of exposure. A definite example of age-related vulnerability is the increased sensitivity of children to psychostimulants, which may exert a small effect on body growth.

In adolescence, long-term risks of certain medications (thyroid and skin effects of lithium, dental caries from anticholinergic agents) can be prevented by alertness to the medical management of the side effects. The risk of unanticipated adolescent pregnancy requires special attention in treatment of girls with lithium (which may cause significant cardiac and other somatic malformations, even with brief exposure during early pregnancy) and certain skin care medications (Accutane).

CONCLUSION

There is a large number of drugs that may potentially influence development. Many of these effects are the progressive result of acute side effects of drugs used in long-term treatments (sedation by phenobarbital interfering with learning and behavior), results of drug intoxication (putative effect of phenytoin on the cerebellum), or consequences of side effects of drugs (skin scarring from acne aggravated by lithium). Appropriate medical management is essential in pediatric pharmacotherapies, and can reduce the impact of this class of "developmental" effects of drugs.

Some age-related effects operate through psychological and social mechanisms: the effect of an infant's arousal and behavior at birth on the parents, or the influence of maternal malnutrition and lack of medical care on recreational drug effects on a fetus.

There are genuine biological examples of age-related toxicological effects on development of the body and brain: psychostimulants (slowing of body growth), aspirin (Reye's syndrome), tetracycline (organ discoloration), and possibly hexachlorophene (impairment of myelin formation) and valproic acid (hepatotoxicity). These effects are exerted through a variety of biological mechanisms.

In this survey of drugs with developmental toxicological effects used in psychiatry, neurology, and medicine, the total number and severity of such effects is perhaps surprisingly low. This may reflect our current state of ignorance or the possibility that physicians (in their urgency for caution or response to uncertainty) may overestimate the frequency of developmental toxicity.

Given the common use of the basic biochemical and physiological mechanisms throughout life, agents that are risky for adults are generally risky for developing organisms as well. Drug trials in adults are often helpful in identifying toxic effects prior to their use in children. If physicians delay the use of "new drugs" in children until there is a history of their use in adults, there will be an opportunity for observing certain toxic effects operating through basic mechanisms. However, there will always be a place for careful initial trials of medications in children for observing possible toxic effects on development.

Among the general principles that emerge in developmental toxicology, it is clear that the effects of drugs on the nervous system are determined not only by dosage and duration, but also by the age of exposure. Early exposure during pregnancy is likely to produce structural changes in the body and brain, whereas later exposure is likely to produce more subtle effects including cognitive and behavioral alterations, particularly inattention and hyperactivity. Some of these effects are self-limited; some are permanent. These effects can be due to single agents, but risks are multiplied when causative factors operate in combination.

Careful empirical studies are needed to distinguish toxic effects induced by drugs from toxic effects induced by the underlying diseases.

Clinicians should maintain a balanced and educated awareness of empirically demonstrated drug effects, continually reexamine patients on long-term medication, and listen carefully to the observations and concerns of children and their parents.

Years or decades will be needed to answer all clinical questions definitively through prospective empirical studies involving infants, children, and adolescents in the course of their psychopharmacologic treatments.

REFERENCES

American Academy of Pediatrics Committee on Drugs: Valproate teratogenicity. Pediatrics 71:980, 1983

American Academy of Pediatrics Committee on Infectious Diseases: Aspirin and Reye's syndrome. Pediatrics 69:810–812, 1982

American Psychiatric Association Task Force on Late Neurological Effects of Antipsychotic Drugs: Tardive dyskinesia. Am J Psychiatry 137:1163–1172, 1980

American Psychiatric Association Task Force on Long-term Effects of Lithium on the Kidney: Report. Washington, DC, American Psychiatric Association (in preparation)

Amsterdam, JD, Winokur A, Caroff S, et al: The effects of desmethylimipramine and lithium on human sperm function. Psychoneuroendocrinology 6:359–363, 1981

Amsterdam JD, Jorkasky D, Potter L, et al: A prospective study of lithium-induced nephropathy: preliminary results. Psychopharmacol Bull 21:81–84, 1985

Apte SN, Langston JW: Permanent neurological deficits due to lithium toxicity. Ann Neurol 13:453–455, 1983

Bacon CJ, Cranage JD, Hierons AM, et al: Behavioral effects of phenobarbitone and phenytoin in small children. Arch Dis Child 56:836–840, 1981

Baier WK, Beck U, Duose H, et al: Cerebellar atrophy following diphenylhydantoin intoxication. Neuropediatrics 15:76–81, 1984

Baldessarini RJ: Drugs used in the treatment of disorders of mood, in The Pharmacological Basis of Therapeutics, 7th ed. Edited by Gilman AG, Goodman LS, Gilman A. New York, Macmillan, 1984, pp 430–434

Baldessarini RJ: Chemotherapy in Psychiatry. Cambridge, Mass, Harvard University Press, 1985

Baldessarini RJ, Cohen BM, Teicher MH: Significance of neuroleptic dose and plasma level in the pharmacological treatment of psychoses. Arch Gen Psychiatry 1987 (in press)

Ballenger CE, Lucke JF, King DW, et al: Cerebellar atrophy in epilepsy and headache: lack of relationship to phenytoin. Neurology 32:910–912, 1982

Bendz H: Kidney function in a selected lithium population: a prospective, controlled, lithium-withdrawal study. Acta Psychiatr Scand 72:451–463, 1985

Bergey GK, Swaiman KF, Schrier BK, et al: Adverse effects of phenobarbital on morphological and biochemical development of fetal mouse spinal cord neurons in culture. Ann Neurol 9:584–589, 1981

Bevelander G, Nakahara H: The effect of diverse amounts of tetracycline on fluorescence and coloration of teeth. J Pediatr 68:114–120, 1966

Caine ED, Margolin DI, Brown GL, et al: Gilles de la Tourette's syndrome, tardive dyskinesia, and psychosis in an adolescent. Am J Psychiatry 135:241–243, 1978

Camfield CS, Chaplin S, Doyle A-B, et al: Side effects of phenobarbital in toddlers: behavioral and cognitive aspects. J Pediatr 95:361–365, 1979

Centers for Disease Control: Reye's syndrome—United States, 1984. Morbidity and Mortality Weekly Report 34:13–16, 1985

Christiansen P, Deigaard J, Lund M: Potency, fertility and sexual hormones in young male epileptics. Ugeskr Laeger 137:2402–2405, 1975

Dalessio DJ: Seizure disorders and pregnancy. N Engl J Med 312:559–563, 1985

Dan BB: Vietnam and birth defects. JAMA 252:936–937, 1984

Davis RE: Manic-depressive variant syndrome of childhood: a preliminary report. Am J Psychiatry 136:702–706, 1979

DeLong GR: Lithium carbonate treatment of select behavior disorders in children suggesting manic-depressive illness. J Pediatr 93:689–694, 1978

Desmond MM, Schwanecke RP, Wilson GS, et al: Maternal barbiturate utilization and neonatal withdrawal symptomatology. J Pediatr 80:190–197, 1972

Dreifuss FE: Fatal liver failure in children on valproate. Lancet 1:47–48, 1987

Dreifuss FE, Santilli N, Menander KB, et al: Valproic acid hepatic fatalities: a retrospective review. Neurology 1987 (in press)

Erickson JD, Mulinare J, McClain PW, et al: Vietnam veterans' risks for fathering babies with birth defects. JAMA 252:903–912, 1984

Ernhart CB, Landa B, Schell NB: Subclinical levels of lead and developmental deficit: a multivariate follow-up reassessment. Pediatrics 67:911–919, 1981

Expert Committee on Pediatric Neurobehavioral Evaluations: Independent Peer Review of Selected Studies Concerning Neurobehavioral Effects of Lead Exposures in Nominally Asymptomatic Children: Official Report of Findings and Recommendations of an Interdisciplinary Expert Review Committee (659-017/7240). Washington, DC, US Government Printing Office, 1983

Feingold BF: Why Your Child is Hyperactive. New York, Random House, 1974

Field TM, Widmayer SM: Developmental follow-up of infants delivered by Cesarean section and general anesthesia. Infant Behavior and Development 3:253, 1980

Fishman MA: Commentary: side effects of phenobarbital. J Pediatr 95:403–404, 1979

Friedman JM: Does Agent Orange cause birth defects? Teratology 29:193–221, 1984

Gelenberg AJ (ed): Psychotropic drugs and the fetus. Biological Therapies in Psychiatry 7:13–14, 1984

Golub MS, Golub AM: Behavioral teratogenesis, in Advances in Perinatal Medicine, Vol 1. Edited by Milunsky A, Friedman EA, Gluch L. New York, Pleneum, 1981, pp 231–293

Gram L, Bentsen KD: Valproate: an updated review. Acta Neurologica Scandinavica 72:129–139, 1985

Gross MD: Growth of hyperkinetic children taking methylphenidate, dextroamphetamine, or imipramine/desipramine. Pediatrics 58:423–431, 1976

Grossman ER, Walchek A, Freedman H, et al: Tetracyclines and permanent teeth: the relation between dose and tooth color. Pediatrics 47:567–570, 1971

Gualtieri CT, Guimond M: Tardive dyskinesia and the behavioral consequences of chronic neuroleptic treatment. Dev Med Child Neurol 23:255–159, 1981

Gualtieri CT, Barnhill J, McGimsey J, et al: Tardive dyskinesia and other movement disorders in children treated with psychotropic drugs. J Am Acad Child Psychiatry 19:491–510, 1980

Gualtieri CT, Quade D, Hicks RE, et al: Tardive dyskinesia and other clinical consequences of neuroleptic treatment in children and adolescents. Am J Psychiatry 141:20–23, 1984

Hanson JW, Buehler BA: Fetal hydantoin syndrome: current status. J Pediatr 101:816–818, 1982

Hanson JW, Myrianthopoulos NC, Harvey MAS, et al: Risks to the offspring of women treated with hydantoin anticonvulsant, with emphasis on the fetal hydantoin syndrome. J Pediatr 89:662–668, 1976

Harley JP, Ray RS, Tomasi L, et al: Hyperkinesis and food additives: testing the Feingold hypothesis. Pediatrics 61:818–828, 1978a

Harley JP, Matthews CG, Eichman P: Synthetic food colors and hyperactivity in children: a double-blind challenge experiment. Pediatrics 62:975–983, 1978b

Hartitzsch B, Hoenich NA, Leigh RJ, et al: Permanent neurological sequelae despite haemodialysis for lithium intoxication. Br Med J 4:757–759, 1972

Heninger GR: Summary recommendations for long-term lithium use, in Continuing Medical Education Syllabus and Scientific Proceedings of the Annual Meeting of the American Psychiatric Association. Washington, DC, American Psychiatric Association, 1984, p 192

Herskowitz J, Rosman NP: Acute hexachlorophene poisoning by mouth in a neonate. J Pediatr 94:495–496, 1979

Herskowitz J, Rosman NP: Autism, schizophrenia, and other psychoses, in Pediatrics, Neurology, and Psychiatry: Common Ground. New York, Macmillan, 1982, pp 97–99

Hill LM, Kleinberg F: Effects of drugs and chemicals on the fetus and newborn. Mayo Clin Proc 53:707–716, 755–765, 1984

Hingson R, Alpert JJ, Day N, et al: Effects of maternal drinking and marijuana use on fetal growth and development. Pediatrics 70:539–546, 1982

Hong CY, Chaput de Saintonge DM, Turner P: The inhibitory action of procaine, (+)propranolol, and (±)propranolol on human sperm motility: antagonism by caffeine. Br J Clin Pharmacol 12:751–753, 1981

Hong CY, Chaput de Saintonge DM, Turner P: Effects of chlorpromazine and other drugs acting on the central nervous system on human sperm motility. Eur J Clin Pharmacol 22:413–416, 1982

Hurwitz ES, Barrett MJ, Bregman D, et al: Public Health Service study on Reye's syndrome and medications. N Engl J Med 313:849–857, 1985

Imbs JL, Danion JM, Welsch M, et al: Renal tolerance of longterm lithium treatment: prospective study on patients suffering from manic-depressive psychosis. Acta Pharmacol Toxicol (Copenh) Suppl 59:161, 1986

Jeavons PM: Non-dose-related side effects of valproate. Epilepsia (Suppl) 25:50–55, 1984

Jefferson JW, Greist JH, Ackerman DL, et al: Lithium Encyclopedia for Clinical Practice, 2nd ed. Washington, DC, American Psychiatric Press, 1987

Jeste DV, Wyatt RJ: Dyskinesias in children and adolescents, in Understanding and Treating Tardive Dyskinesia. New York, Guilford Press, 1982, pp 171–177

Johnson GFS, Hunt GE, Duggin GG, et al: Renal function and lithium treatment: initial and follow-up tests in manic-depressive patients. J Affective Disord 6:249–263, 1984

Jones KL, Smith DW: Recognition of the fetal alcohol syndrome in early infancy. Lancet 2:999, 1973

Kargas GA, Kargas SA, Bruyere HJ, et al: Perinatal mortality due to interaction of diphenhydramine and temazepam. N Engl J Med 313:1417–1418, 1985

Keepers GA, Clappison VJ, Casey DE: Initial anticholinergic prophylaxis for acute neuroleptic induced extrapyramidal syndromes. Arch Gen Psychiatry 40:1113–1117, 1983

Kraemer HC, Korner A, Anders T, et al: Obstetric drugs and infant behavior: a reevaluation. J Pediatr Psychol 10:345–353, 1985

Krigman MR, Bouldin TW, Mushak P: Lead, in Experimental and Clinical Neurotoxicology. Edited by Spencer PS, Schaumburg HH. Baltimore Williams & Wilkins Co, 1980, pp 490–507

Lafferman JA, Silbergeld E: Erythrosin B inhibits dopamine transport in rat caudate synaptosomes. Science 205:410–412, 1979

Lambrou DB, Tahos BS, Lambrou KD: In vitro studies of the phenomenon of tetracycline incorporation into enamel. J Dent Res 56:1527–1532, 1977

Lammer EJ, Chen DT, Hoar RM, et al: Retinoic acid embryopathy. N Engl J Med 313:837–841, 1985

Lemoine P. Harousseau H, Borteyru J-P, et al: Les enfants des parents alcooliques: anomalies observees, a propos de 127 cas. Arch Fr Pediatr 15:830–831, 1968

Levin RM, Amsterdam JD, Winokur A, et al: Effects of psychotropic drugs on human sperm motility. Fertil Steril 36:503–506, 1981

Lindstedt G, Nilsson L-A, Walinder JA, et al: On the prevalence, diagnosis and management of lithium-induced hypothyroidism in psychiatric patients. Br J Psychiatry 130:452–458, 1977

Lindvall O, Nilsson B: Cerebellar atrophy following phenytoin intoxication. Ann Neurol 16:258–260, 1984

Lustig FW: A fatal case of hexachlorophene ("pHisoHex") poisoning. Med J Aust 50:737, 1963

Madsen JR, Campbell A, Baldessarini RJ: Effects of prenatal treatment of rats with haloperidol due to altered drug distribution in neonatal brain. Neuropharmacology 20:931–939, 1981

Mattes J, Gittelman-Klein R: A crossover study of artificial food colorings in a hyperkinetic child. Am J Psychiatry 135:987–988, 1978

Mattes JA, Gittelman R: Growth of hyperactive children on maintenance regimen of methylphenidate. Arch Gen Psychiatry 40:317–321, 1983

Melgaard B: The neurotoxicity of ethanol. Acta Neurol Scand 67:131–142, 1983

Moffet HL: Pediatric Infectious Diseases: A Problem-Oriented Approach. Philadelphia, JB Lippincott Co, 1975, pp 463–464

Monson RR, Rosenberg L, Hartz SC, et al: Diphenylhydantoin and selected congenital malformations. N Engl J Med 289:1049–1052, 1973

Morrell P, Sutherland GR, Buamah PK, et al: Lithium toxicity in a neonate. Arch Dis Child 58:539–541, 1983

Mortensen PB: Inhibition of fatty acid oxidation by valproate. Lancet 2:856–857, 1980

Needleman HL, Gunnoe C, Leviton A, et al: Deficits in psychologic and classroom performance of children with elevated dentine lead levels. N Engl J Med 300:689–695, 1979

Nicholi AM: The nontherapeutic use of psychoactive drugs. N Engl J Med 308:925–933, 1983

Nora JJ, Nora HA, Toews WH: Lithium, Ebstein's anomaly, and other congenital heart defects. Lancet 2:594–595, 1974

Nurnberg HG, Prudic J: Guidelines for treatment of psychosis during pregnancy. Hosp Community Psychiatry 35:67–71, 1984

O'Connell CM, Fried PA: An investigation of prenatal cannabis exposure and minor physical anomalies in a low risk population. Neurobehav Toxicol Teratol 6:345–350, 1984

Ouibell EP: The thalidomide embryopathy: an analysis from the U.K. Practitioner 225:721–726, 1981

Paulson GW, Paulson, RB: Teratogenic effects of anticonvulsants. Arch Neurol 38:140–143, 1981

Perrild H, Hegedus L, Arnung K: Sex-related goitrogenic effect of lithium carbonate in healthy young subjects. Acta Endocrinol 106:203–208, 1984

Platt JE, Campbell M, Green WH, et al: Cognitive effects of lithium carbonate and haloperidol in treatment-resistant aggressive children. Arch Gen Psychiatry 41:657–662, 1984

Polizos P, Engelhardt DM, Hoffman SP, et al: Neurological consequences of psychotropic drug withdrawal in schizophrenic children. Journal of Autism and Childhood Schizophrenia 3:247–253, 1973

Popper C: Child and adolescent psychopharmacology, in Psychiatry. Edited by Michels R, Cavenar JO, Brodie HKH, et al. Philadelphia, JB Lippincott Co, 1985

Powell-Jackson PR, Tredger JM, Williams R: Hepatotoxicity to sodium valproate: a review. Gut 25:673–681, 1984

Rapoport JL, Mikkelsen EJ, Werry JS: Antimanic, antianxiety, hallucinogenic and miscellaneous drugs, in Pediatric Psychopharmacology: The Use of Behavior Modifying Drugs in Children. Edited by Werry JS. New York, Brunner/Mazel, 1978, pp 316–355

Reynolds EH: Mental effects of antiepileptic medication: a review. Epilepsia (Suppl) 24:85–95, 1983

Rimmer E, Richens A: An update on sodium valproate. Pharmacology 5:171–184, 1985

Rogers MF, Schonberger LB, Hurwitz ES, et al: National Reye's syndrome surveillance, 1982. Pediatrics 75:260–264, 1985

Rosenberg L, Mitchell AA, et al: Lack of relation of oral clefts to diazepam use during pregnancy. N Engl J Med 309:1282–1285, 1980

Rosengarten H, Friedhoff AJ: Enduring changes in dopamine receptor cells of pups from drug administration to pregnant and nursing rats. Science 203:1133–1135, 1979

Rosenstein SN: Disorders of the teeth and supporting structure, in Pediatrics, 17th ed. Edited by Rudolph AM, Hoffman JIE. Norwalk, Connecticut, Appleton-Century-Crofts, 1982, pp 878–879

Rothner AD: Valproic acid: a review of 23 fatal cases. Ann Neurol 10:287, 1985

Rutter M: Raised lead levels and impaired cognitive/behavioural functioning: a review of the evidence. Dev Med Child Neurol (Suppl) 22:1–25, 1980

Safer D, Allen R, Barr E: Depression of growth in hyperactive children on stimulant drugs. N Engl J Med 237:217–220, 1972

Scanlon JW, Hollenbeck AR: Neonatal behavioral effects of anesthetic exposure during pregnancy, in Advances in Perinatal Medicine, Vol 3. Edited by Milunsky A, Friedman EA. New York, Plenum, 1983, pp 165–203

Schapiro MB, Rosman NP, Kemper TL: Effects of chronic exposure to alcohol on the developing brain. Neurobehav Toxicol Teratol 6:351–356, 1984

Schmidt D: Adverse effects of valproate. Epilepsia (Suppl) 25:44–49, 1984

Schooler NR, Kane JM: Research diagnoses for tardive dyskinesia. Arch Gen Psychiatry 39:486–487, 1982

Schou M, Goldfield MD, Weinstein MR, et al: Lithium and pregnancy: I. report from the register of lithium babies. Br Med J 2:135–136, 1973

Schultz FR, Hayford JT, Wolraich ML, et al: Methylphenidate treatment of hyperactive children: effects on the hypothalamic-pituitary-somatomedin axis. Pediatrics 70:987–991, 1982

Schwachman H, Schuster A: The tetracyclines in applied pharmacology. Pediatr Clin North Am 3:295–303, 1956

Selevan SG, Lindbohm ML, Hornung, RW, et al. A study of occupational exposure to antineoplastic drugs and fetal loss in nurses. N Engl J Med 313:1173–1178, 1985

Shaywitz SE, Cohen DJ, Shaywitz BA: Behavior and learning difficulties in children of normal intelligence born to alcoholic mothers. J Pediatr 96:978–982, 1980

Shaywitz SE, Hunt RD, Jatlow P, et al: Psychopharmacology of attention deficit disorder: pharmacokinetic, neuroendocrine, and behavioral measures following acute and chronic treatment with methylphenidate. Pediatrics 69:688–694, 1982

Shiono PH, Mills JL: Oral clefts and diazepam use during pregnancy. N Engl J Med 311:919–920, 1984

Silverstein FS, Parrish MA, Johnston MV: Adverse behavioral reactions in children treated with carbamazepine (Tegretol). J Pediatr 101:785–787, 1982

Singer I, Rotenberg D: Mechanisms of lithium action. N Engl J Med 289:254–260, 1973

Smigan L, Bucht G, Von Knorring L, et al.: Longterm lithium treatment and renal functions: a prospective study. Neuropsychobiology 11:33–38, 1984

Snyder SH, Reynolds IJ: Calcium-antagonist drugs: receptor interactions that clarify therapeutic effects. N Engl J Med 313:995–1002, 1985

Soyka LF, Joffe JM: Male mediated drug effects on offspring. Prog Clin Biol Res 36:49–66, 1980

Spencer PS, Schaumburg HH: Classification of neurotoxic disease: a morphological approach, in Experimental and Clinical Neurotoxicology. Edited by Spencer PS, Schaumburg HH. Baltimore, Williams & Wilkins Co, 1980, pp 92–101

Starko KM, Ray CG, Dominquez LB, et al: Reye's syndrome and salicylate use. Pediatrics 66:859–864, 1980

Sterman AB, Schaumburg HH: Neurotoxicity of selected drugs, in Experimental and Clinical Neurotoxicology. Edited by Spencer PS, Schaumburg HH. Baltimore, Williams & Wilkins Co, 1980, pp 593–612

Stores G: Behavioural effects of anti-epileptic drugs. Dev Med Child Neurol 17:647–658, 1975

Suzuki K: Special vulnerabilities of the developing nervous system to toxic substances, in Experimental and Clinical Neurotoxicology. Edited by Spencer PS, Schaumburg HH. Baltimore, Williams & Wilkins Co, 1980, pp 48–61

Swaiman KF, Neale EA, Schrier BK, et al: Toxic effect of phenytoin on developing cortical neurons in culture. Ann Neurol 13:48–52, 1983

Swanson JM, Kinsbourne M: Food dyes impair performance of hyperactive children on a laboratory learning test. Science 207:1485–1487, 1980

Tarsy D, Baldessarini RJ: Tardive dyskinesia. Annu Rev Med 35:605–623, 1984

Tarsy D, Baldessarini RJ: Clinical and pathophysiological features of movements disorders induced by psychotherapeutic agents, in Movement Disorders. Edited by Donald A, Shah N. New York, Plenum, 1986, pp 365–389

Tein I, MacGregor DL: Possible valproate teratogenicity. Arch Neurol 42:291–293, 1985

Thurston JH, Hauhart RE: Chronic valproate induces key enzymes of hepatic fatty acid oxidation and ketogenesis in infant mice. Pediatr Res 1987 (in press)

Towfighi J: Hexachlorophene, in Experimental and Clinical Neurotoxicology. Edited by Spencer PS, Schaumburg HH. Baltimore, Williams & Wilkins Co, 1980, pp 440–455

Trimble M: Anticonvulsant drugs, behavior, and cognitive abilities. Curr Dev Psychopharmacol 6:65–91, 1981

Tuchmann-Duplessis H: Influence of certain drugs on the prenatal development. Int J Gynaecol Obstet 8:777–797, 1970

Van Thiel DH, Ross GT, Lipsett MB: Pregnancies after chemotherapy of trophoblastic neoplasms. Science 169:1326–1327, 1970

Vestergaard P, Amdisen A: Lithium treatment and kidney function: a follow-up study of 237 patients in long-term treatment. Acta Psychiatr Scand 63:333–345, 1981

Vorhees CB, Brunner RL, Butcher RE: Psychotropic drugs as behavioral teratogens. Science 204:1220–1225, 1979

Weiss B, Williams JH, Margen S, et al: Behavioral responses to artificial food colors. Science 207:1487–1489, 1980

Weyman J, Porteous JR: Tetracycline discoloration and bands in human teeth: report of a case. Br Dent J 115:499–502, 1963

White SW, Besanceney C: Systemic pigmentation from tetracycline and minocycline therapy. Arch Dermatol 119:1–2, 1983

Wilson N, Forfar JC, Godman MJ: Atrial flutter in the newborn resulting from maternal lithium ingestion. Arch Dis Child 58:538–539, 1983

Winder C, Kitchen I: Lead neurotoxicity: a review of the biochemical, neurochemical and drug induced behavioural evidence. Prog Neurobiol 22:59–87, 1984

Wolf SM, Forsythe A: Behavior disturbance, phenobarbital, and febrile seizures. Pediatrics 61:728–731, 1978

Woody JN, London WL, Wilbanks GD: Lithium toxicity in a newborn. Pediatrics 47:94–96, 1971

Yakovlev PI, Lecours A-R: The myelogenetic cycles of regional maturation of the brain, in Regional Development of the Brain in Early Life. Edited by Minkowski A. Oxford, Blackwell, 1967

Zackai EH, Mellman WJ, Neiderer B, et al: The fetal trimethadione syndrome. J Pediatr 87:280–284, 1975

Zafrani ES, Berthelot P: Sodium valproate in the induction of unusual hepatotoxicity. Hepatology 2:648–649, 1982

Zimmerman HJ, Ishak KG: Valproate-induced hepatic injury: analysis of 23 fatal cases. Hepatology 2:591–597, 1982

Chapter 5

Medical Unknowns and Ethical Consent: Prescribing Psychotropic Medications for Children in the Face of Uncertainty

Charles Popper, M.D.

Chapter 5

Medical Unknowns and Ethical Consent: Prescribing Psychotropic Medications for Children in the Face of Uncertainty

As psychiatrists use more psychopharmacological treatments for children and adolescents, we are faced with making clinical decisions in an area of medicine with many scientific unknowns: biochemical development of the brain and possible critical periods of vulnerability, changes in the pharmacokinetic handling of drugs in children during growth, age-related shifts in the pharmacodynamic response of different body systems during maturation, and long-term effects of drugs on the body and brain resulting from medication use during adolescence and childhood.

This book has reviewed a wide range of scientific unknowns regarding the techniques, safety, and long-term effects of one of our most powerful psychiatric treatment modalities for children.

This chapter explores the effects of incomplete medical knowledge on treatment decisions by physicians and patients. For the physician, ethical and medical judgments are required for making decisions about the use of new treatments for childhood disorders, possible special risks to children of medications that have primarily been used in adults, relative risks of drug treatments and disease processes, and the concept of treatment safety in this era of probabilistic thinking in medicine. For the patient, "informed consent" provided by the family and "assent" provided by the child may fulfill current legal requirements, but still be clinically insufficient. To achieve ethical

Thanks are due to J. Andrew Billings, M.D., Tim Clancy, Rose Demeo, Seymour Kety, M.D., and Arthur Rosenberg, Esq., for their balance, vision, and experience.

consent, it is necessary for the physician to follow and respond to the child's and parents' development of understanding.

This is not a comprehensive review of all ethical issues in psychiatry. There are many ethical issues raised by psychiatric diagnosis and treatment, the right to choose treatment or nontreatment, informed consent, therapeutic coercion, experimentation, and training (Bloch and Chodoff 1984; Edwards 1982; Kentsmith et al. 1986; Rosenbaum 1982). In child and adolescent psychiatry, these issues are further complicated by the additional dimensions of developmental changes in cognitive capacities, by parents and physicians making decisions for children, and by intrafamilial splitting of consent decisions (Graham 1984; Morrissey et al. 1986). In child and adolescent psychopharmacology, the frequent use of "empirical trials" in actual practice blurs the distinction between clinical experimentation and medical treatment.

This chapter focuses on two aspects of ethical decision making that commonly have a direct and clear effect on the prescribing habits of practicing physicians: how to justify psychopharmacological treatments of children when the effects of these biological therapies in adolescents and children are at present largely unknown, and how to obtain ethical consent by the child and family for these treatments.

Making Medical Decisions Today

Until future developmental pharmacoscientific research has provided clarification, clinicians of today need to treat a generation of adolescents and children with our present knowledge. We do not know how current decisions to use or withhold medication (or any psychiatric treatment, for that matter) will be viewed in the future. To use or not use medication—either can be an error, when viewed in retrospect.

For now, medical decisions are based on evaluating two sets of incomplete medical knowledge: information regarding toxic effects of drugs and information regarding toxic effects of diseases.

To ask only, "What do we know? . . . Do we know enough about the effects of this drug in a child?" is to ask a purely academic question. We need to ask also, "What are the effects of the psychiatric disorder on this child?"

Weighing the Unknowns: Risks of Drugs and Risks of Diseases

Psychotropic medications are not prescribed to healthy children. Medications are used in "trade-off" for the management of the child's presenting problems, diseases, and disorders. By looking at medication decisions for a developmental or childhood-onset disorder as evaluating a trade-off, we encounter a second set of unknowns: What are the long-term developmental effects of the disease?

In child psychiatry, as in psychiatry in general, we unhappily do not yet know of the long-term effects of the diseases we are treating. Our science barely allows us to differentiate the various disorders encountered clinically in psychiatry. It will be decades before follow-up studies can delineate the long-term psychiatric course, medical consequences, and psychosocial effects transmitted to the next generation.

Consider the example of lithium. What are the chances that the side effects and unknown adverse effects of a drug like lithium will be more risky than lithium-responsive conditions of childhood? At this time, we know little about the effects of lithium in children. But we also know quite little about the natural course of the illness of lithium-responsive conditions in children.

We do know that, in adults, manic-depressive illness is associated with a 15 percent mortality from suicide alone, and that morbidity and mortality due to concomitant cardiovascular and other medical illnesses are also high (Avery and Winokur 1976).

We do not yet have adequate follow-up data on lithium-responsive childhood disorders (with or without treatment). However a possibly useful general principle that is emerging in the study of childhood biopsychiatric diseases is that the early-onset illnesses are more severe than adult-onset disorders. For major depression (Carlson 1984, Kovacs et al. 1984), dysthymia (Kovacs et al. 1984), and other major adult disorders, the appearance in childhood of a typically adult disorder often signals a more severe disease and a more troubled course.

If 15 percent of adult manic-depressives end their lives in suicide, it is reasonable to predict that the outlook for childhood-onset conditions will be no better.

Do we believe that lithium will produce 15 percent mortality in child and adolescent lithium-responsive patients?

A major concern about lithium is the potential for renal damage with long-term use. Recent prospective studies of kidney effects of lithium have reduced initial concerns (see Chapter 4). These better-controlled studies show minor effects on renal structure and generally insignificant functional changes (American Psychiatric Association Task Force on Long-term Effects of Lithium on the Kidney 1987). Since early exposure and treatment duration might be factors in the appearance of the renal changes, the introduction of lithium therapy in children may speculatively involve an increased risk. Separate evaluation of the lithium effects on kidney function in children will be required.

We may have other medical concerns about lithium: risks of undercorrection of thyroid effects of lithium in growing children and seriously scarring acne in adolescents. These problems can be adequately managed if appropriately monitored.

Even if future pharmacological data show that lithium has unexpected effects, including serious physical developmental effects, our best medical judgment at this time would be that it seems unlikely that lithium use in children would produce dangers comparable to a 15 percent premature death rate. It seems unlikely that this drug, even with undetermined long-term effects, will be more dangerous than such a biopsychiatric disorder.

The clinician is still faced with the question of whether the symptomatic severity in an individual is sufficient to warrant drug treatment during childhood, whether other clinical variables permit safe administration of medication to the child, whether psychotropic treatment should be deferred until a particular phase of the illness (e.g., until a period of high risk for fatal self-destructive behavior), or whether drug treatment during childhood improves the subsequent course of illness, help-seeking, or development. Apart from these major clinical issues, the more limited pharmacological question concerns balancing the risk of the drug and the risk of the disease.

Another example is provided by the anxiety disorders. Panic disorder was initially viewed as an uncomfortable but not dangerous disease in adults. Yet adults with panic disorder have a 20 percent mortality from suicide and a twofold increase in deaths due to diseases of the circulatory system (Coryell et al. 1982). There are no available medical follow-up data on children and adolescents with panic disorder, but it is not credible that antidepressants in children might be more harmful than a 20 percent suicide rate.

Again, this example requires a weighing of unknowns (including the assumption that antidepressants reduce suicide). However, reasonable medical judgment would place greater odds on the relative safety of this drug treatment compared to this disease process.

Take a different case of an anxious and withdrawn child, with chronic underachievement and poor self-confidence, who responds to antidepressant medication. Compared with more disturbed children, this child might be viewed as having a "good prognosis" with a reasonable chance at satisfactory adjustment in future employment and socialization. For this latency-age child with major depression, we may not see the one-in-three risk of the child developing a conduct disorder and growing into a life of delinquency or social marginality (Puig-Antich 1982). Again, we must balance the unknown risks of a course of antidepressants against the dangers of consequences such as these.

The medical data required for ethical decisions are not only pharmacological: To make these clinical judgments, it is essential to have a knowledge of the consequences of the medical disorders. Until we have the basic knowledge of the natural course of child and adolescent psychiatric conditions, we cannot know whether it is safer to use or not to use a drug.

There is a need for follow-up studies regarding the large array of psychiatric disorders treated with psychotropic medications in children (Table 1).

Multiyear and multidecade follow-up studies of the natural course of child and adolescent psychiatric conditions requires a type of personal commitment and institutional financing that is new in psychiatry. To secure this type of information, we need governmental grants that are structured across decades, and private institutions supporting programs for follow-up research, as well as individual clinician-researchers in psychiatry and child psychiatry who are willing to stay with a project as a stable part of their careers.

Age-Dependent Toxicity of Five Clinically Used Drugs

Looking outside of psychiatry at all the drugs used over the years in medicine, few medications that are safe in adults have unsafe effects on the maturational process in children. It will always be necessary to test established drugs used by adults in separate clinical trials for children to determine safety. Also, it will always be necessary to test for teratogenic effects because the intrauterine period is known to be a special case of uniquely high developmental vulnerability. However, for drugs known to be safe in adults, once developmental pharmacokinetic factors regarding dosage regimens are understood, it is not very likely that a pharmacodynamic danger will be uncovered or that critical developmental damage will occur—apart from the period of intrauterine vulnerability.

At this time, there are only three medications that are established to be generally safe in adults but unsafe in children over age 3: tetracyclines, psychostimulants, and aspirin. The tetracyclines have been found to produce dental (and other organ) discoloration in children under 8 years of age, a significant cosmetic effect that would probably be tolerated if there were not an abundance of alternative antibiotics available. Psychostimulants produce some growth retardation, but the effect appears to be slight—influencing less than 2 percent of the variance in adult height outcome (Mattes and Gittelman 1983)—an acceptable risk in view of the known psychodevelopmental consequences of attention deficit-hyperactivity disorder (Weiss and Hechtman 1986). The third example is the

Table 1. Current and Changing Indications for Psychopharmacological Treatment in Children

Category	Established	Probable	Conjectural
Psychostimulants	Attention deficit-hyperactivity disorder (ADHD)		Conduct disorder Behavioral impulsivity Emotional lability Inattentiveness
Antidepressants	ADHD Enuresis	Separation anxiety disorder Panic disorder Anorexia nervosa Bulimia nervosa Major depression School phobia Some conduct disorder* Some phobic disorders*	Behavioral impulsivity Emotional lability Inattentiveness
Neuroleptics	Overt psychosis Tourette's disorder Unmanageable behavior Aggression Destructiveness Agitation Self-mutilation ADHD	Behavioral impulsivity Autistic disorder Pervasive developmental disorders Head-banging Major anxiety	

Lithium	Bipolar I disorder	Bipolar II disorder Recurrent depressive disorders Rage outbursts* Conduct disorder*	Cyclothymic disorder Aggressivity Behavioral impulsivity*
Antianxiety Agents	Sleep walking Night terrors Anxiety disorders Minor anxiety Anticipatory Situational Presurgical Seizures Localized muscle spasm Sleep induction	Tics Head-banging Body-rocking	Conduct disorder Behavior disorders
Antihistaminic/ Antimuscarinic Agents	Sleep induction Agitation		Minor anxiety*
Anticonvulsants	Seizure/behavioral disorders	Affective disorders Unipolar* Bipolar*	Behavioral disorders Rage outbursts
Clonidine		Tourette's disorder	ADHD*
Propranolol		Rage outbursts Anxiety	
Naltrexone		Autistic disorder*	Pervasive developmental disorder*

*These are recent changes. Compare to Popper (1985).

involvement of aspirin in the development of Reye's syndrome, an uncommon but potentially fatal hepatic and neurological compli-cation. Again, the availability of an alternative medication (acet-aminophen) eliminates this clinical problem in most cases. If alter-native antipyretics were not available, it is probable that the low risk of this fatal condition would be considered acceptable as a trade-off in many cases where symptomatic control of fever was judged clin-ically valuable.

A fourth example, valproic acid, is less clearly documented. This anticonvulsant appears to have a greater risk of leading to hepatotoxic metabolite formation in children than in adults (Dreifuss 1987). Valproate-induced hepatotoxicity is the most serious example of idio-syncratic metabolic hypersensitivity in children, potentially proceed-ing to acute liver failure, and, in some cases, death.

Valproic acid has a novel chemical structure, a branched-chain fatty acid, which is unique among commercially available drugs in the United States. Since its introduction in the United States in 1978 (Europe in 1968), case reports of fatal hepatotoxicity appeared in 1979, and studies describing over 60 cases were reported by 1982 (Rothner 1985; Zafrani and Berthelot 1982; Zimmerman and Ishak 1982).

If there is confirmation of an increased risk in children, it is plau-sible that an age-related vulnerability in fatty acid metabolism may be involved. Particularly in view of the increased susceptibility of children to defects of mitochondrial fatty acid-metabolizing enzymes (including Reye's syndrome), this risk may reflect a newly uncovered metabolic problem related to fatty acid structures (Mortensen 1980; Thurston and Hauhart 1987; Zimmerman and Ishak 1982).

Unlike psychostimulants, aspirin, and tetracycline, the toxic effect of valproic acid is also seen occasionally in adults. If valproic acid had been initially introduced for treating adults, there would probably have been evidence of the valproate hepatotoxicity and the need for monitoring of liver function tests prior to its introduction for chil-dren. Further, its novel chemical structure should remind us that clinical use of a substantially innovative chemical agent should be delayed in children until there have been at least several years of clinical use in adults.

A fifth agent, hexachlorophene, raises a developmental concern primarily for premature and very young infants. Heavy exposure through bathing and high absorption through skin may lead to in-creased toxicity, which includes a developmental effect on myelin formation. This agent does not appear to present a significant risk to children subsequent to early infancy, and so is not directly relevant to the vulnerability of children who may be candidates for psycho-pharmacological treatment.

Of all the drugs used throughout medicine, these five medications are the prime examples of drugs whose safety in children would not be adequately predicted from clinical treatment of adults or laboratory studies in animals.

Drugs Shown Safe in Adults: Implications for Adolescents and Children

There is a common belief that the safety of drugs in children is a totally separate matter from the safety of drugs in adults. However, for the vast majority of drugs used in medicine, adult safety usually implies safety for children and adolescents.

To base all future medical judgments on the thalidomide disaster, one of the many intrauterine toxins, is clouded medical judgment. There are many drugs with major developmental effects during this critical developmental phase. The intrauterine period is a critically vulnerable phase in development, which is empirically quite different from the postuterine period from birth to age 3 years, and is surely the wrong model for judgments made for children older than age 3 years.

For clinical use of psychotropic medication in children and adolescents, it is appropriate to follow early clinical research, particularly concerning the pharmacokinetic handling of drugs in children. Pending the outcome of such research, the best working model for understanding the effect of medications in children and adolescents is the adult model, not the intrauterine model.

Wait for a Track Record in Adults

A track record in adults is still desirable prior to the use of new medications in children. It is not advisable to use new drugs that are just being introduced into commercial availability. A new antidepressant or neuroleptic agent that has fewer side effects than older medications may be introduced, but may well be found to have side effects that were not anticipated in the early field trials. Such unexpected side effects typically emerge during the first few years of use in the adult population. It required about 1 to 4 years of general clinical use in the United States to recognize the seizures produced by maprotiline, the persistent penile erections produced by trazodone, the hematological effects of nomifensine, or the tardive dyskinesia of neuroleptics.

Optimally, to uncover adverse effects, it would be helpful to wait until several million adults were treated with a new medication, and there were clinical trials and pharmacokinetic studies in children, before a new drug becomes used routinely in children.

In practice, this optimal situation may take many years. In cases where older medications have failed, clinicians often use a new drug "for the benefit of the individual" before these studies are complete.

There are no governmental or established clinical guidelines for the introduction of new medications in children. Physicians' judgments are influenced by the state of the medical literature on the use of a particular drug in adults and children, and by the clinical circumstances of the individual patient. Depending on the specific situation, it may be prudent to wait perhaps 3 to 5 years for a minor chemical innovation (a new analogue of a commercially available drug already in use for some years), or 10 to 15 years before using a new category or class of pharmacological agents in children.

This degree of caution does not remove the risk, especially if direct studies on children are not yet reported. However, once a drug is known in adults for some years, for the vast majority of agents used in medicine, the medical odds are good that the medication will be safe and the side effects similar (or predictable) in children and adolescents in general.

It is not always necessary to wait for a track record in adults before introducing "new" drug treatments for children. If a psychotropic drug has major technical advantages over previous treatments (an uncommon occurrence), or if a serious illness has limited alternative treatments (e.g., fenfluramine or naltrexone therapy of autism), then the rapid introduction of "new" drugs may be advisable with the understanding that clinical safety has not received prior evaluation.

This assertive use of new psychopharmacological treatments for children and adolescents is a recent development in psychiatry.

Other Scientific Unknowns Regarding Children

If psychiatry ever comes to provide pharmacological treatments to children under age 3 as a matter of routine, a different level of clinical and scientific knowledge regarding pharmacology will be needed. There are many factors during the first 3 years of life that are substantially different from later childhood and adulthood, and that introduce exceedingly complex technical problems into early pediatric treatment (Morselli 1977). Pharmacokinetic factors change rapidly during the first 3 years, with different parameters moving at their own speed and in varying directions. Smaller body compartments require precise dose measurements and timing. Metabolic hypersensitivity of the liver is far greater and unpredictable.

As an aside, there are other types of scientific unknowns regarding children and adolescents that may modify the clinical practice of drug use in psychiatry. We cannot infer that a neurobiological diagnostic test that is valid in adults will be diagnostically valid in children. There are many tests in neurology and medicine for which the establishment of ranges of normal and pathological "cut-off" values cannot be extended to adolescents and children. For example, if the dexamethasone suppression test (DST) were established as clinically useful in adults, its clinical utility, diagnostic cut-off values, and dosage and timing (based on developmental pharmacokinetics) would need to be determined separately in adolescents and children. Alternately, it is possible that the DST may turn out to have more clinical value in children (where identification of major depression on clinical grounds is often difficult) than in adults. Similarly, therapeutic plasma levels of antidepressants, which may be metabolized in children by developmentally changing enzyme systems and may display age-specific metabolite profiles, need to be separately described for different age groups.

Studying Drug Effects While Studying Disease Effects

Three drugs with known developmental effects in post-toddlers (tetracycline, stimulants, and aspirin) had been in use in millions of children before their developmental side effects were uncovered. Psychostimulants were in use for more than 30 years before the effect on height was found, and more than a decade was required to delineate the small magnitude of this effect. Yet tooth color and body size are as easily observed and objectively quantitated as any measure in biology. Less obvious effects, such as changes in affect or cognition, may take much longer to find.

Even if such subtle effects are identified, they may be tolerated in exchange for control over suicidality, psychosis, or major affective or cognitive abnormalities, particularly if the drug treatment enhances special education, psychotherapy, or developmental progress.

The delineation of more mild and subtle drug effects will require clinical research focusing on developmental changes in adolescents and children already receiving pharmacological treatments. To find possible mild or subtle developmental drug effects, the research will need to be done simultaneously with use in clinical treatments.

Data on drug effects will be collected in the future—at the same time that we collect data on disease effects. Until then, we will not "know" the relative safety of drugs and diseases, and our judgments in clinical practice will be largely based on the traditions of our training and past experience, and biased by our personal response to unknowns.

Illusion of Safety in the Familiar

For now, we will remain subject to the "illusion of safety in the familiar," a psychological bias familiar to decision analysts who empirically observe human response to risk (Nelkin and Brown 1984).

We are subject to an illusion of perceiving safety in these familiar diseases, which may seem "more safe" than the unfamiliar drug treatments. Even for biopsychiatric illness, we may be inclined to underestimate and underperceive their major morbidity and mortality. Especially when dealing with a specific case, we may "accept" the risks of familiar disorders.

When discussing relatively unfamiliar drug treatments, one often hears the alternative suggestion of using older and more "conventional" therapies. "Why not use psychotherapy or a behavioral treatment to deal with child and adolescent disorders? We at least know they are safe, and won't produce body damage." The impression of safety of "conventional" therapies exemplifies the "illusory sense of safety in the familiar."

We do not have a carefully developed science of the risks of psychotherapy: of negative therapeutic reactions, of withdrawal (termination) effects, or of dependency complications—and even less is known in adolescents and children. We, in fact, know little about the relative safety of the various treatment modalities.

The problem of concurrent treatment and research does not pertain exclusively to pharmacotherapy. The relative safety and value of all treatment modalities will be determined alongside each other in the future. With all treatments, we will operate at the clinical level without essential empirical information to guide us to statistically maximal "safety." Yet familiarity may lead us to see illusory safety—and to under-perceive the actual morbidity and mortality of illnesses under conventional treatment approaches.

FDA Guidelines for Drug Advertisements Do Not Regulate Clinical Practice

There is also another common clinical approach: "The Food and Drug Administration (FDA) can tell us when a commercial drug has been sufficiently tested to use with children. The manufacturers run clinical field trials that test the safety and efficacy of new drugs in children, and the FDA issues guidelines for their use. Until they have approved a drug, it is unwise to experiment." Yet the FDA guidelines are meant to regulate the advertising of pharmaceutical houses, not the clinical practice of physicians. The regulations are designed for drug manufacturers, not for physicians or patients.

The FDA itself has emphasized this point, asserting:

> Under the Federal Food, Drug, and Cosmetic Act, a drug approved for marketing may be labeled, promoted, and advertised by the manufacturer only for those uses for which the drug's safety and effectiveness have been established and which the FDA has approved. . . . The [Food, Drug, and Cosmetic] Act does not, however, limit the manner in which a physician may use an approved drug. Once a product has been approved for marketing, a physician may prescribe it, for uses or in treatment regimens or patient populations that are not included in approved labeling. . . . Accepted medical practice often includes drug use that is not reflected in approved drug labeling. (Department of Health and Human Services 1982)

The phrase "for uses or in treatment regimens or patient populations" acknowledges physicians' discretion regarding indications (diagnosis or symptom), doses, and age groups.

FDA guidelines are not designed to describe optimal care of patients. The FDA in 1987 still directed advertising to indicate a maximum imipramine dose of 2.5 mg/kg for children, even though medical resources were often recommending doses up to 5.0 mg/kg (with electrocardiographic monitoring) as an appropriate dose for depressed children.

Sometimes physicians feel bound by FDA guidelines for defensive legal reasons: "Even if the FDA is not regulating clinical practice, the *Physicians' Desk Reference* (PDR) is viewed as an authoritative legal source. If a problem came up, an opposing lawyer would certainly cite the FDA guidelines to imply that a physician was acting unwisely in using a drug outside of 'approved' age limits." It is important to know that there is legal recognition of the physician's and patient's rights to make decisions based on individual clinical situations. It is wise to cite a textbook chapter (Popper 1985) or reference book (Campbell et al. 1985; Wiener 1985) in the patients' medical records to support use outside of approved "labeling," but it is not generally essential to inform a family when clinical use does not conform to advertising regulations.

Decision Making in Probabilistic Situations

We have all grown into our profession through medical training, which emphatically taught us to "First, do no harm." This dictum grows out of an early era in medicine predominated by medicinal toxins and lotions. In the primitive climate of early medical practice, limiting professional harm was a major life-saving measure.

In the modern world of "statistical medicine," with complex diagnostic systems, layers of treatment, and partial understanding of the inherent risks of natural course and interactive benefits of multimodal intervention programs, we are required to use probabilistic assessments and thoughtful decision analysis (Bursztajn et al. 1981).

Ethical treatment will increasingly entail a more complex dictum than "Do no harm." If our first dictum is caution, then it may be understood in our modern age as advising thoughtfulness regarding decision making, not as withholding responses in the face of medical unknowns.

Consent and the Capacity to Evaluate Complexity

As decision analysis in medicine and psychiatry becomes more probabilistic, we face new problems in our still-developing science of informed consent. We can explain to parents that psychopharmacological treatment of adolescents and children is still emerging, that diagnostic indications are not precise, and that our understanding of long-term side effects is incomplete. We can describe the serious risks and uncertainties regarding the long-term course of illness. We can state that our understanding of drug-related effects and disease-related effects is insufficient to say with certainty which approach provides greater safety. We can also inform them that we typically use drugs whose effects are well known in adults, and that there are few drugs in medicine that are known to be safe in adults but unsafe in children.

Yet this is quite an extraordinarily complex set of concepts for a parent to evaluate. What are the chances that the child's caretaker will be able to assess fully this series of statistically qualified statements? Can logic of this type be articulated in the ordinary clinical setting in an effective manner? Do parents who only partially grasp this complex piece of thinking become unable to provide "informed" consent?

ETHICAL CONSENT

Given the unknowns in child psychopharmacological treatment, the physician may find it unusually challenging to ask for consent for treatment. Some of these difficulties derive from the medical unknowns, but some derive from the nature of informed consent.

Both informed consent laws and clinical techniques are themselves only partially developed and continue to evolve as we practice (Miller 1980). As a clinical/ethical/legal expectation, the concept of informed consent is incomplete and unclear, and introduces its own uncertainties into the clinical setting.

Informed consent concepts, both legal and clinical, will be reviewed, with particular attention to adolescent and child psycho-pharmacological treatment. A protocol for obtaining and documenting both legal and clinical consent will be outlined.

"Good Enough" Consent

What level of "informed consent" currently operates clinically in our routine psychiatric practice: in our university and teaching hospitals (where we do not routinely tell patients who the trainees are), or in private offices? Do we, as guardians of our profession as well as of patients, operate with "full" informed consent in our routine clinical practice?

We typically accept a degree of informed consent as satisfactory to proceed with a treatment. Typically, the parents understand some things about the risks of a medical treatment, but do not know other things. They may have been told, but forgot (Jaffe 1981; Meisel and Roth 1983). How many side effects can a patient remember? A level of detail may be clinically judged too much for a parent to absorb at the particular time. We are often satisfied simply to get "enough" permission to proceed with a treatment. Particularly in psychiatry, we accept varying degrees of cognitive and affective support for a treatment as the natural circumstances in which treatments proceed.

How often have you had a bright and educated patient listen to a few minutes of a treatment description, and then simply say, "Whatever you think is best, doctor." The patient who turns the decision back to you is avoiding dealing emotionally with the complexity of the situation.

The parents who say "Do whatever you think is best" may appear to give the kind of support that we seek for a treatment. Bringing a child into therapy for weekly meetings, and on time, may be viewed as good support.

Is this "good enough" consent?

We have only a few studies in psychiatry concerning the degree of informed consent provided in actual clinical settings by patients or patients' parents (Meisel and Roth 1981). We have virtually no studies regarding adolescents and children.

In the major empirical study of informed consent in adult psychiatry, Lidz et al. (1984) found little evidence that informed consent law or policy is operational in routine practice. Patients often did not want to be their own primary decision makers, doctors did not disclose information freely, and responsibility often "floated" between caretakers. Yet the authors' subjective sense was that generally decisions were being made responsibly by both physicians and patients.

We take this acquiescence in real-life clinical situations as effective consent: "good enough" to proceed with treatment. We recognize that it is legitimate clinical practice to deal with ambivalence and reluctance regarding receiving help or treatment as a part of the treatment process—as we go along with the treatment.

Informed Consent: The Legal Concept

Acquiescent consent is "legal" if it fulfills the basic legal criteria of informed consent. In child and adolescent psychiatric treatment, and in medical practice generally, the patient (or child's parent) is provided:

1. the purpose of the treatment (benefits)
2. a description of the treatment process (including procedure, duration, and costs)
3. an explanation of the risks of the treatment (with an estimate of their probability); that is,
   a) risks that would ordinarily be described by psychiatrists (the standard of practice); and/or
   b) risks relevant to making the decision (material risk), even if not routinely described by most psychiatrists
4. a statement of the alternatives to the proposed treatment, including nontreatment (their purposes, risks, and processes)

These four elements are expected to be delivered verbally, although some hospitals and even some state laws require the supplementary use of written consent for certain treatments (e.g., surgery and electroconvulsive therapy, which involve anesthesia and temporary life support). A clear exception pertains in emergencies, for which there is a legally recognized physician's prerogative to proceed with needed treatment without consent, although contact with the family is expected once possible. A second exception is "therapeutic privilege": a physician may withhold information viewed as detrimental (physically or psychologically) to the patient. Other departures from these principles have been discussed, such as the possibility of deferred consent (Abramson et al. 1986).

Especially for novel child and adolescent psychopharmacological treatments, a fifth component of informed consent may be considered:

5. an explicit statement that there may be *unknown* risks of these drugs

This warning is relevant for any drug treatment, but is particularly appropriate when developmental dimensions are added to the set of unknowns.

Physicians may hesitate to state this medical unknown with explicitness. However, it may be easier to be explicit if unknowns about the drug are communicated in a balanced way along with unknowns about the disease.

Since children are generally unable to give legally valid "informed consent" in their own behalf, parents become legally responsible for making these "consent" judgments for them.

There is no consensus regarding a particular age at which children become competent to provide informed consent. Various legal decisions have been based on the medical situation, life circumstances, family factors, and developmental capacities (Langer 1984). There is increasing recognition of cognitive and judgmental capacities of children, and of legal rights of children to make certain decisions for themselves regarding surgery, medical treatment, abortion, and organ donation. There are differences in state laws and in regional practices (Holder 1985; Morrissey et al. 1986). The U.S. Supreme Court has not supported the notion of a fixed age of competence below the age of majority (age 18 to 21, depending on state law). Courts as well as clinicians appear inclined to let individual circumstances determine the age of medical consent. There are recognized "shadings" in the legal age of medical consent, but consent itself is not viewed in shades.

From a legal point of view, consent is either provided or it is not. There is no recognition of "in between" states of ambivalence, partial understanding, cognitive styles, intrapsychic defenses, or "becoming" informed during the course of treatment. Ambivalent consent is legally adequate so long as the parent or patient agrees after being "informed" of the purpose, risks, process, and alternatives. At the present state of development of the informed consent law, what is required legally is the physician's disclosure, not the parents' understanding or lack of ambivalence. A consent may be sufficient for legal purposes, but not for clinical purposes.

Emotional Consent: A Clinical Concept

The need for "emotional consent" goes beyond legal requirements: It is crucial for clinical care. Aside from whatever information may be provided, the child and parents must emotionally "come to terms" with the nature of the child's illness and the treatment recommendations.

For the parents, the drug treatment of a child may imply a different or more serious problem than they suspected. The nature of the illness may be viewed in terms of how long the drug will be used and whether the symptoms might return after drug administration is stopped. The recommendation to use a drug may require parents to integrate new knowledge and to "wrestle" emotionally with the decision to accept medical treatment.

Bypassing or speeding through this clinical process leaves parents only partially (or compliantly) prepared to support the treatment of the child. In some cases, it may be useful to delay treatment until the parents can do their best in grappling with the questions generated by a treatment recommendation—especially if the disease concept requires understanding both biological and psychological aspects of the child's condition and future. It is helpful to provide a specific model of how the mind and body interact to produce the symptoms (Popper and Famularo 1983), especially when the psychotherapy and drugs are used in combination to treat a biopsychiatric disorder.

Assent of the Child

Children are generally unable to provide legal consent, so the principle of "assent" has been developed. Children can contribute substantially to the consent process, even though it may not be the legal equivalent of informed consent.

The use of assent is a sensible clinical step that helps parents and physicians be aware of the doubts and beliefs of the child. Obtaining assent implies that a child will be given attention, provided information, and offered a chance to express feelings about the treatment.

The child's ideas about medication may include fears about "being crazy," mind control, personal weakness, dependency, life-long use, passivity, weakness, being poisoned, hangovers, sterility, or over-excitation. Alternately, magical expectations or excessive hopes about the medication may interfere with a realistic attitude about the treatment. These fantasies about pills usually reflect covert but similar resistances to other aspects of the treatment, and to receiving help in general. Pills are a concrete form of help. Drug therapy can expose and clarify the child's dynamics of getting and using help.

At what age should assent be obtained? A child's assent for participation in medical research is advised at age 7 years (National Commission for the Protection of Human Subjects of Biomedical and Behavioral Research 1978). This recommendation is derived partly from common law, which traditionally views age 7 as the "age of discretion." Modern cognitive psychology has been cited as support for this benchmark (Koocher 1981). Children would not be able to discuss their motivations or conceptualize long-term consequences prior to the Piagetian stage of concrete operations.

Periodic reevaluation of assent may be helpful. As a child develops, new capacities for understanding may alter earlier impressions and judgments. A child may come to regret a previous decision, or may renew a formerly acquiescent decision with deeper understanding and autonomy. Particularly for children or adolescents on long-term drug treatments, it is helpful to provide periodic opportunities for updating their information load and emotional involvement.

Parental Consent for a Child's Treatment

In addition to the ethical and legal questions that arise when treatment decisions are made by a parent for a child (Graham 1984), clinical problems arise if parents disagree about treatment. A child's resistance to a treatment may be based on stated or unverbalized doubts of a parent—even if that parent is separated from the family and living far away. A parent's reluctance may be based on reasonable opinion, but may also reflect an inability to see the child's problem or accept help, an expression of hostility at the child, or oppositional splitting with the other parent. Until substantive approval for treatment is received from both parents (sometimes requiring separate discussions with the physician), a child may lack the necessary parental support. It is unreasonable to expect a child to take a medication comfortably when even one parent does not back the treatment.

In child and adolescent psychopharmacological treatment, it is common for one or both parents to have a related genetic biopsychiatric illness. When a parent providing consent is preoccupied or psychologically symptomatic (anxious, depressed, psychotic), questions may arise at certain times about the legitimacy of their consent for the child's treatment. Some psychotic patients may not understand information regarding treatment consent, even if they subjectively feel that they understand (Irwin et al. 1985). However, a parent may be psychiatrically impaired but remain competent to give consent for a child's treatment. In these circumstances, though, intuitive doubts about the parents' judgment may influence the child's comfort in accepting a treatment. In extreme situations, a guardian (relative or adult friend) may be needed to provide the child with a clear sense of caretaker consent. The handling of the parents' consent is an essential feature of the clinical management of the child.

Clinical problems may also arise when the child and parents disagree about the need for a treatment. In rare cases, a child's solo decision to decline medication treatment is nonoppositional and rational. Typically, however, if a child refuses medication despite parental support, there is often a more general pattern of oppositional interaction within the family, and the child may feel or actually be forced to take the medication. Therapeutic coercion places the child in a passive and nonresponsible position. The legality of therapeutic coercion is uncertain, and clinically the treatment must then deal with the child's anger at the coercion. When possible, it is usually better to address the child's psychodynamic needs, mobilize parental rewards (parents' attention, time, and praise) to counter the oppositionalism, and work with the child's refusal of medication as a concrete example of the child's refusal to receive help. Therapeutic coercion is often a part of the psychiatric treatment of children, but it may be inadvisable for nonestablished drug treatments.

Similarly, "instant consent" to treatment—whether child's or parents'—is based on compliance rather than consent. This procedure fails to address their genuine questions (regarding the disorder, treatment, and prognosis), reduces effective support for treatment, and increases the risk of the child or family stopping the medication in midtreatment. The best time for dealing with resistance to medication is at the start of treatment, not after the passive "compliance" breaks down.

Yet, like adults, child and adolescent patients may not want to make their own treatment decisions, and may prefer their caretakers to use their parental and professional judgments. In such cases, they may want to be "informed" enough to know what to expect, not to make decisions (Annas et al. 1977; Strull et al. 1984). For these individuals, "good enough consent" may entail knowing what is likely to happen during a treatment—what is predictable, not what is unknown. This kind of knowing enhances the capacity to cope with bad outcomes, and may be important to the patient's sense of self-control. In some instances, lacking this coping strategy may be more upsetting than a negative treatment outcome.

Documenting Consent

For adult patients, the use of a signed consent form appears to indicate that the patient has provided informed consent, but the presence of the signature does not certify that the patient has understood, remembered, or cared. The signature proves only that the patient was present in the room.

To be useful from a legal point of view, consent forms need to be specific (Miller 1980). Generalized or vague written consent forms have not fared well as evidence in courts, unless the language is explicit and shows what kind of information was disclosed. Written material alone is insufficient: The courts expect that information is also provided verbally and understandably. Signed consent forms have legal value mainly in the extreme event that a patient claims that no consent was sought.

Such consent forms do not relieve the physician of responsibility, or protect the child from potential pharmacological risks, and certainly do not substitute clinically for good verbal explanations or the opportunity to ask questions of the prescribing physician (Munetz and Roth 1985; Vaccarino 1978).

Although a signed consent form may appear to provide formalized consent, a more clinically relevant approach involves the physician's documented description of the consent process: who was involved, how did the child participate, were the decision makers preoccupied by other matters, did they seem to understand the nature of the treatment, did they ask questions that suggested good understanding of the potential risks, did they seem to listen, what behavioral and affective reactions were observed, was there confusion or difficulty in understanding certain points, was there an interest in hearing detail, did the patient want to make the decision, did the parents want the physician to make the decision for them?

From a legal point of view, much of this information cannot be safely placed in a patient's medical record. It could increase potential legal liability to document that the consent was based on less than full information, received ambivalent support, or was subject to further discussion.

Nonetheless, documentation of consent and assent is useful clinically at the start of treatment, and for subsequent follow-up of the developing understanding and continuing consent.

Figure 1 provides a model form that can be used to document the start of a child's psychopharmacological treatment, including some general aspects of consent and assent for the patient's medical record. The medical documentation should include: (1) diagnoses; (2) specific target symptoms; (3) drug regimen; (4) concurrent medications (and anticipated drug interactions); (5) neurological and medical disorders (and possible interactions with the medication); (6) possible risks of medication abuse; and (7) statement of informed consent, including the degree of detail regarding risks, process, and alternatives (e.g., state some specific risks) plus the general level of awareness of individuals in the consent interviews.

Figure 2 can be used to document the physician's view of the "degree" of understanding held by patient and parents at the start of treatment. This is "legally sensitive" data, and so should be maintained separately from the patient's record. Such sensitive but clin-

Figure 1. Documentation for Initiation of Psychopharmacological Treatment of Child

Child _____

Psychiatrist _____ **Date** _____

Drug Treatment
  Psychostimulant _____ Neuroleptic _____
  Antidepressant _____ Anticonvulsant _____
  Lithium _____ Antianxiety _____ Other _____

Drug Name _____

Regimen Starting dose _____

  Body weight _____ Height _____ **Age** _____

  Anticipated rate of increase _____

  Approximate top dosage _____

Justification
  _____ Medication is likely to be helpful.
  _____ Low likelihood of help, but
          trial is warranted by severe illness.
  _____ Symptoms are mild, but risk/benefit is favorable.
  _____ Treatment is novel (risk/benefit is uncertain), but severity of illness
          warrants drug trial.

Diagnosis

  Axis 1 _____

  Axis 2 _____

  Axis 3 _____

Features of: 0 = absent   1 = some/slight   2 = present
  _____ Affective disorder
  _____ Hallucinations or delusions
  _____ Loss of reality sense
  _____ Attention deficit disorder/hyperactivity
  _____ Anxiety disorder (separation, phobic, panic)
  _____ Other anxiety
  _____ Other impulsivity
  _____ Other: _____

Figure 1. Documentation for Initiation of Psychopharmacological
Treatment of Child   *(continued)*

Target Symptoms for Medication
_____ Psychosis (overt hallucination or delusion)
_____ Loss of reality sense
_____ Depressive affect
_____ Suicidality: _____ ideation _____ action
_____ Impulsivity: _____ ideation _____ action
_____ Violence: _____ ideation _____ action
_____ Self-harm: _____ ideation _____ action
_____ Anger: _____ ideation _____ action
_____ Rituals/obsessions
_____ Phobic symptoms
_____ Panic episodes
_____ Separation anxiety
_____ Other anxiety (not anxiety disorder)
_____ Hyperactivity
_____ Inattentiveness
_____ Sleep disruption
_____ Slow morning arousal
_____ Appetite excess
_____ Appetite lack
_____ Cognitive distortion

Other Current Medications
(Indicate anticipated or potential drug interactions)

_____

_____

_____

Neurological Evaluation
Work-up included: neurological exam ____ EEG ____ CT ____

Positive findings that might relate to drug treatment
_____ seizure disorder
_____ abnormal EEG without "seizure disorder"
_____ abnormal CT
_____ soft neurological signs
_____ physical anomalies (e.g., dysmorphic face)
_____ dyskinesias or tics
_____ other: _____

Do neurological findings warrant a special warning regarding drug-induced
seizures?   Yes _____ No _____

Figure 1. Documentation for Initiation of Psychopharmacological Treatment of Child   *(continued)*

Medical Evaluation
Work-up included: physical exam, height, weight _____
CBC, blood profile, urinalysis _____
liver function tests _____ thyroid screen _____
EKG _____ creatinine _____
other lab tests _____

Positive findings which might relate to drug treatment
_____ cardiac abnormality
_____ liver
_____ kidney
_____ asthma
_____ hypertension
_____ thyroid
_____ other

Risk of Medication Abuse
_____ Substance abuse   by patient _____ parent _____ sibs _____
_____ Suicidal use   by patient _____ parent _____ sibs _____
_____ Self-medication   by patient _____ parent _____ sibs _____
_____ Accidental ingestion by young sibs
_____ Inconsistent administration or inadequate supervision at home

Information Provided for Consent and Assent

Information	Information was provided to		
Purpose (benefits)	patient _____	mother _____	father _____
Risks (dangers)	patient _____	mother _____	father _____
Process (what to expect)	patient _____	mother _____	father _____
Alternative treatments	patient _____	mother _____	father _____

Specify some of the risks discussed (to suggest level of detail)

_____

_____

Figure 1. Documentation for Initiation of Psychopharmacological Treatment of Child   *(continued)*

Caretakers' consent is judged sufficient for legal purposes

Mother's consent   yes _____ no _____ unavailable _____

Father's consent   yes _____ no _____ unavailable _____

Guardian's consent   yes _____ no _____ unavailable _____

  Specify guardian _____

Child's role in decision process

  Consented _____ Assented _____ Too young to assent _____

---

ically relevant data may include the amount of information that was not disclosed, the level of understanding communicated by questions asked by patient or parents, the physician's working impression of the parents' mental competence to provide consent, a sense of the amount of information that the parents could accept, the degree of emotional and intellectual involvement of parents and child in the process, and doubts regarding general quality of the consent and assent at the time of starting treatment. Figure 2 might be kept by a physician to follow clinical status, used in clinical supervision in a teaching hospital, or reviewed by a quality care team monitoring consent in a hospital. An alternative approach has been proposed: administering a questionnaire or written test to the patient as a part of the consent process to demonstrate their degree of understanding (Miller and Willner 1974).

The advisability of withholding such clinical information from a medical record underscores the incompleteness of informed consent concepts and laws. The current laws effectively require secrecy to maintain the split between legally acknowledged and unacknowledged aspects of this clinical procedure. However, the strength of these laws rests in their providing societal guidance for the physician to place essential information into the hands (and hopefully the minds) of the patient and family.

Ethical Consent and Medical Unknowns

A primary purpose of informed consent is to provide a basic minimum of control, or opportunity for control, to the patient. As Ingelfinger (1972) said, "The deceptions of the past are no longer tolerated."

Figure 2.   Quality Review of Consent for Psychopharmacological
Treatment of Child

(Do not place this form in patient's medical records.)

Child _____

Psychiatrist _____ **Date** _____

Drug Treatment
  Psychostimulant _____ Neuroleptic _____
  Antidepressant _____ Anticonvulsant _____
  Lithium _____ Antianxiety _____ Other _____

Drug Name _____

Urgency at Start of Treatment
  _____ Routine
  _____ Emergency, but full consent was obtained prior to treatment
  _____ Due to emergency, full consent was not obtained prior to treatment

Parental Consent obtained by

	Interview	Phone	Via spouse	Not available
Mother	_____	_____	_____	_____
Father	_____	_____	_____	_____
Guardian	_____	_____	_____	_____

Parental Competence to Consent at Start of Drug Treatment
  _____ Both parents are competent to provide consent for this
    treatment.
  _____ Mother _____ or Father _____ may be not competent for this
    consent:
    _____ Documented in chart.   _____ Not yet documented.
  _____ Consent provided by guardian

Parental Consent at Start of Drug Treatment	Mother	Father
Total time of consent discussion was		
less than 10 minutes.	_____	_____
less than 30 minutes.	_____	_____
less than 50 minutes.	_____	_____
more.	_____	_____

Figure 2. Quality Review of Consent for Psychopharmacological
Treatment of Child   *(continued)*

Discussion included full disclosure of information regarding
    major acute side effects.   ⎯⎯⎯   ⎯⎯⎯
    all long-term side effects.   ⎯⎯⎯   ⎯⎯⎯
    possibility of unknown effects.   ⎯⎯⎯   ⎯⎯⎯
    alternative treatments.   ⎯⎯⎯   ⎯⎯⎯
Degree of informational understanding is
    excellent.   ⎯⎯⎯   ⎯⎯⎯
    incomplete but substantial.   ⎯⎯⎯   ⎯⎯⎯
    limited.   ⎯⎯⎯   ⎯⎯⎯
Emotional involvement in decision making
    is full.   ⎯⎯⎯   ⎯⎯⎯
    was avoided and, in effect, turned over to
        physician.   ⎯⎯⎯   ⎯⎯⎯
    was compliant with spouse's stronger preference.   ⎯⎯⎯   ⎯⎯⎯
Process of consent involved the parent asking
    few or no questions.   ⎯⎯⎯   ⎯⎯⎯
    questions that revealed confusion and
        misunderstanding.   ⎯⎯⎯   ⎯⎯⎯
    questions revealing good understanding.   ⎯⎯⎯   ⎯⎯⎯
Explanations (value, risks, side effects) will
        probably be
    nearly fully remembered.   ⎯⎯⎯   ⎯⎯⎯
    require subsequent repetition.   ⎯⎯⎯   ⎯⎯⎯
    poorly retained.   ⎯⎯⎯   ⎯⎯⎯
At start of treatment, overall quality of consent is
    ⎯⎯⎯ excellent.
    ⎯⎯⎯ adequate, given clinical limitations.
    ⎯⎯⎯ limited, but sufficient to begin treatment.

Child's Assent at Start of Drug Treatment
    ⎯⎯⎯ Participatory and supportive.
    ⎯⎯⎯ Limited understanding, but accepting and cooperative.
    ⎯⎯⎯ Doubtful or ambivalent, but reluctantly acquiescent.
    ⎯⎯⎯ Opposed, but compliant to parental directives.
        ["therapeutically coerced"]
    ⎯⎯⎯ Other (Please specify): ⎯⎯⎯⎯⎯⎯⎯⎯⎯⎯⎯⎯⎯⎯⎯⎯⎯⎯⎯

Note. This form is not to be placed in the patient's medical chart. It may
be used for personal or supervisory review, or sent to the hospital monitor
of quality of care.

If "full" informed consent will be given, at best, by only a fraction of parents at the start of a treatment, "consent" will probably exceed the cognitive capacity of virtually all adolescents and children. Their "assent" to treatment will signify mainly their sense of personal self-control and self-determination in the process rather than an informed understanding of the probabilistic issues involved. Younger children will want to know mainly the color of the pills and their size, and perhaps about their taste. Slightly older children may want to know when they will take them and whether they have to take them. These children will generally not be concerned, or ask questions, about the safety of the pills. Adolescents will have difficulty judging what lies ahead in their future, colored by their ongoing learning about their place in the world, and have limited ability to gauge the unknowns of their disease-related future.

As we enter an age of increasingly complex decision analysis and probabilistic thinking in medicine, we may eventually reach a point

Figure 3. Some Recommendations for Obtaining Consent

1. Discuss directly with the patient and each parent.
2. Look for indications that the person understands. (Separate meetings may help you focus on each person.)
3. Give time for questions.
4. Continue the discussion at least until the person's responses indicate that they know what to expect in the process of the treatment.
6. Determine if the patient is able to know more than what to expect.
7. Inform openly. Do not minimize or withhold risks.
8. Be explicit about uncertainty. (Discuss unknowns about drugs and diseases together, to maintain a sense of clarity of purpose.)
9. Do not overwhelm with excess information at one sitting.
10. Use multiple visits to reinform and reclarify: Informed consent is a process.
11. Tell the patient what to do if they run into a problem with the drug (especially a big problem).
12. If emergency management is needed and there is no time to obtain consent, inform the family as soon as possible.
13. Follow the pattern of information and emotional processing. Use it as a model for understanding other aspects of the patient's coping style and help-seeking.
14. Write a note in the medical record about the consent. Document general descriptors of the patient's involvement (attentiveness) and specific examples of warnings (to indicate level of detail discussed).
15. If a signed consent form is used, make it specific about what the patient is being told.
16. The goal is to provide understanding and appropriate hope.

where the cognitive requirements for making treatment decisions will exceed all but a few of our consenting patients and their parents. As we approach this era, we will need to learn more about how articulately to describe factors relevant to treatment decisions (Benson 1984; Brown and Funk 1986; Diamond 1985; Grundner 1980; Gutheil et al. 1984; Johnson et al. 1986; Mathews 1983; McNeil et al. 1982).

Epstein and Lasagna (1969) showed that consent forms can easily overload an adult's cognitive capacities, and that a patient may understand more about a drug's effects if told less information rather than given all relevant information.

As we integrate these now-classic findings, we need to think more precisely about how to present information for these medical decisions for effective understanding by our patients—children and adults—in a manner that respects their individuality and that empirically optimizes their control.

Psychiatry and medicine will remain a science of individuals, guided by generalizations but with treatment decisions being made by a clinician for the benefit of an individual. Already our treatments are largely based on "partial information" and "effective acquiescence." The ethical use of psychopharmacological treatments in children depends on the physician's ability to conceptualize drug-related and disease-related effects, to make judgments in the face of medical unknowns, to articulate complex decision-related facts, and to maintain an assertive clarity in guiding treatments that support and strengthen a patient's capacity for independence and self-reliance.

CONCLUSION

Psychiatrists searching for improved treatments for children and adolescents are beginning to bring the products of the biological psychiatry movement into clinical practice. Potential age-specific and developmental dangers of psychotropic medications become a significant concern. Past experience in medicine has yielded five clinically used drugs with age-specific or long-term developmental toxicity. Tetracycline (discoloration of teeth and other organs), aspirin (Reye's syndrome), and psychostimulants (growth slowing) are established examples. Valproic acid (hepatotoxic metabolite formation) probably also represents a risk, but the vulnerability is not definitely greater in children than adults. Hexachlorophene is primarily a risk for young infants, and is probably not a major risk for older children—at ages when they may be candidates for psychopharmacological treatment. Valproic acid, aspirin, and hexachlorophene toxicities are seen at any age to some degree, and might have been anticipated if a track record in adults was available prior to their use in children.

It is generally advised that, for psychiatric treatment of children and adolescents, drugs be introduced after safety is first determined in adults: Wait 3 to 5 years for minor chemical innovations before using a newly available drug in children (and perhaps 10 to 15 years for a substantially new chemical structure), unless compelling clinical reasons make it advisable to proceed despite a lack of prior experience in adults.

There is only a small number of drugs that present significant development-related or age-specific risks after the extreme vulnerability to teratological effects during the intrauterine period. For most drugs used in medicine, an agent that is safe in adults is likely to be safe in children. The best working model for children of age 3 to 16 years is the adult model, not the intrauterine model.

It will also be helpful to follow pediatric pharmacokinetic and pharmacodynamic research. Dosage regimens need to be adjusted for age as well as body size. Pharmacodynamic studies of short-term side effects in children may also modify use (e.g., increased parkinsonian and dystonic motor reactions of neuroleptics).

Certain age-specific developmental effects result from short-term drug side effects that have not received appropriate medical management. For example, lithium may aggravate acne in adolescents and may cause skin scarring if not adequately treated. Antidepressants and other psychotropic agents have anticholinergic side effects that cause dry mouth; if not properly managed by ordinary oral hygiene, certain cases may show increased caries formation and perhaps long-term effects on dental development. In chronic treatments, the acute effects of sedating drugs may have cumulative or progressive influences on learning if excessive sedation is not corrected. The class of "cumulative" developmental drug effects can be avoided by proper medical management of standard side effects.

There may also be unknowns among the acute side effects of medications. An acute but as yet unknown side effect of a drug may contribute to the appearance of this cumulative type of long-term developmental toxicity.

Pharmacokinetic and pharmacodynamic studies will always have a place in child and adolescent psychiatry.

At present, psychopharmacological treatment of children under 3 years old is best avoided. Pharmacokinetics in children before age 36 months is enormously complex, well studied in pediatrics, and quite different from older children and adults. In the future, psychiatrists will require specialized knowledge and consultation to use medications in this age range. Indications for the use of psychotropic agents are being currently described in older children and are quite rudimentary in preschool children. Drug treatment of very young children may be justified only in special and extreme circumstances.

Even for older children and adolescents, psychopharmacological treatment entails biological risks that are only partially known. However, the childhood biopsychiatric illnesses entail developmental risks (underachievement, conduct disorder, drug abuse, suicide) that are also partially undefined.

The relative developmental risks of drugs and diseases require empirical evaluation, alongside the variety of psychiatric treatment modalities. Follow-up studies that compare the effects of psychotropic medications, other psychiatric treatments, and untreated course of illness will be needed before medical treatments can be judged on secure grounds.

Follow-up studies on the many child and adolescent psychiatric disorders may take decades to amass. Until such data are collected starting in the youths themselves, treatment preferences will be influenced by training, past experience, "adult" psychiatric thinking, and physicians' personal capacity for unbiased decision making in the face of unknowns.

The physician will form professional judgments regarding treatment decisions based on medical education opportunities, the medical literature, and clinical consultation with specialists. The FDA, which regulates the commercial advertising of drugs, places no limits (age, diagnosis, or dose) on the physicians' and patients' clinical decisions. Despite the unknowns, we know enough now to guide much clinical practice in child and adolescent psychopharmacology.

Comfortable use of these medications depends on physicians' knowhow in obtaining the ethical involvement of the patient and family in consenting to these treatments. The value of signed consent forms is limited by the common inability of adults to absorb information on highly detailed documents. Descriptions of parental consent and child's assent discussions cannot be placed undiluted into a patient's medical documents because current legal standards do not recognize "partial" informed consent or emotional ambivalence. Informed consent law and policy is incomplete and unclear, similar to various aspects of the psychiatric pharmacosciences of children and adolescents. The physician is left to personal judgment in managing these basic problems in obtaining ethical consent.

Consent for treatment is an ongoing process of reeducating and reevaluating during the course of illness and growth. A consent may be sufficient for legal purposes, but not for patients.

To parents, how do we usefully present unknowns about drugs and diseases in children? How do children actually participate in a consent process? How do we respond to the changing indications for psychotropic drugs in children? What is "good enough" consent in these settings?

The process of obtaining informed consent for these treatments makes these ambiguities "public."

The problems are not avoided by letting children grow into adulthood before using psychopharmacological treatments. For major psychiatric disorders in childhood, not using drugs is not the same as doing no harm.

Despite the concerns regarding long-term risks, the assertive use of drugs can be developmentally protective.

There is no end point or completion date for development. At no point in life does an organism become immune to the long-term effects of drugs—or illnesses.

REFERENCES

Abramson NS, Meisel A, Safar P: Deferred consent: a new approach to resuscitation research on comatose patients. JAMA 255:2466–2471, 1986

American Psychiatric Association Task Force on Long-term Effects of Lithium on the Kidney: Report. Washington, DC, 1987 (in preparation)

Annas GJ, Glantz LH, Katz BF: The current status of the law of informed consent to human experimentation, in Informed Consent to Human Experimentation: The Subject's Dilemma. Cambridge, Mass, Ballinger, 1977, pp 27–61

Avery D, Winokur G: Mortality in depressed patients treated with electroconvulsive therapy and antidepressants. Arch Gen Psychiatry 33:1029–1037, 1976

Benson PR: Informed consent: drug information disclosed to patients prescribed antipsychotic medication. J Nerv Ment Dis 172:642–653, 1984

Bloch S, Chodoff P (eds): Psychiatric Ethics. New York, Oxford University Press, 1984

Brown P, Funk SC: Tardive dyskinesia: barriers to the professional recognition of an iatrogenic disease. J Health Soc Behav 27:116–132, 1986

Bursztajn H, Feinbloom RI, Hamm RM, et al: Medical Choices, Medical Chances: How Patients, Families, and Physicians Can Cope with Uncertainty. New York, Delacorte Press, 1981

Campbell M, Green WH, Deutsch SI: Child and Adolescent Psychopharmacology. Beverly Hills, Calif, Sage Publications, 1985

Carlson GA: A comparison of early and late onset adolescent affective disorder. Journal of Operational Psychiatry 15:46–50, 1984

Coryell W, Noyes R, Clancy J: Excess mortality in panic disorder: a comparison with primary unipolar depression. Arch Gen Psychiatry 39:701–703, 1982

Department of Health and Human Services, United States Government: Use of approved drugs for unlabeled indications. FDA Drug Bull 12:4–5, 1982

Diamond R: Drugs and the quality of life: the patient's point of view. J Clin Psychiatry 46:29–35, 1985

Dreifuss FE, Santilli N, Menander KB, et al: Valproic acid fatalities: a retrospective review. Neurology, 1987 (in press)

Edwards RB (ed): Psychiatry and Ethics. Buffalo, Prometheus Books, 1982

Epstein LC, Lasagna L: Obtaining informed consent. Arch Intern Med 123:682–688, 1969

Graham P: Ethics and child psychiatry, in Psychiatric Ethics. Edited by Bloch S, Chodoff P. New York, Oxford University Press, 1984

Grundner TM: On the readability of surgical consent forms. N Engl J Med 302:900–902, 1980

Gutheil TG, Bursztajn H, Brodsky A: Malpractice prevention through the sharing of uncertainty: informed consent and the therapeutic alliance. N Engl J Med 311:49–51, 1984

Holder A: Legal Issues in Pediatrics and Adolescent Medicine. New Haven, Yale University Press, 1985

Ingelfinger FJ: Informed (but uneducated) consent. N Engl J Med 287:465–466, 1972

Irwin M, Lovitz A, Marder SR, et al.: Psychotic patients' understanding of informed consent. Am J Psychiatry 142:1351–1354, 1985

Jaffe R: Informed consent: recall about tardive dyskinesia. Compr Psychiatry 22:434–437, 1981

Johnson MW, Mitch WE, Sherwood J, et al: The impact of a drug information sheet on the understanding and attitude of patients about drugs. JAMA 256:2722–2724, 1986

Kentsmith DK, Salladay SA, Miya PA (eds): Ethics in Mental Health Practice. Orlando, Fla, Grune & Stratton, 1986

Koocher GP: Competence to consent: psychotherapy, in Children's Competence to Consent. Edited by Melton GB, Koocher GP, Saks MJ. New York, Plenum, 1981

Kovacs M, Feinberg TL, Crouse-Novak MA, et al.: Depressive disorders in childhood, 1: a longitudinal prospective study of characteristics and recovery. Arch Gen Psychiatry 41:229–237, 1984

Langer DH: Medical research involving children: some legal and ethical issues. Baylor Law Review 36:1–39, 1984

Lidz CW, Meisel A, Zerubavel E, et al: Informed Consent: A Study of Decisionmaking in Psychiatry. New York, Guilford Press, 1984

Mathews JJ: The communication process in clinical settings. Soc Sci Med 17:1371–1378, 1983

Mattes JA, Gittelman R: Growth of hyperactive children on maintenance regimen of methylphenidate. Arch Gen Psychiatry 40:317–321, 1983

McNeil BJ, Pauker SG, Sox HC, et al.: On the elicitation of preferences for alternative therapies. N Engl J Med 306:1259–1262, 1982

Meisel A, Roth LH: What we do and do not know about informed consent. JAMA 246:2473–2477, 1981

Meisel A, Roth LH: Toward an informed discussion of informed consent: a review and critique of the empirical studies. Arizona Law Review 25:265–346, 1983

Miller LJ: Informed consent. JAMA 244:2100–2103, 2347–2350, 2556–2558, 2661–2662, 1980

Miller R, Willner HS: The two-part consent form: a suggestion for promoting free and informed consent. N Engl J Med 290:964–966, 1974

Morrissey JM, Hofmann AD, Thrope JC: Consent and Confidentiality in the Health Care of Children and Adolescents: A Legal Guide. New York, Free Press, 1986

Morselli PL (ed): Drug Disposition During Development. New York, Spectrum Publications, 1977

Mortensen PB: Inhibition of fatty acid oxidation by valproate. Lancet 2:856–857, 1980

Munetz MR, Roth LH: Informing patients about tardive dyskinesia. Arch Gen Psychiatry 42:866–871, 1985

National Commission for the Protection of Human Subjects of Biomedical and Behavioral Research: Protection of human subjects: research involving children: report and recommendations. Federal Register 43:2084–2114, 1978

Nelkin D, Brown MS: Taking risks. Transaction/Social Science and Modern Society 21:43–47, 1984

Popper C: Child and adolescent psychopharmacology, in Psychiatry. Edited by Michels R, Cavenar JO, Brodie HKH, et al. Philadelphia, JB Lippincott Co, 1985

Popper C, Famularo R: Child and adolescent psychopharmacology, in Developmental-Behavioral Pediatrics. Edited by Levine MD, Carey WB, Crocker AC, et al. Philadelphia, WB Saunders Co, 1983, p 1157

Puig-Antich J: Major depression and conduct disorder in prepuberty. J Am Acad Child Psychiatry 21:118–128, 1982

Rosenbaum M (ed): Ethics and Values in Psychotherapy. New York, Free Press, 1982

Rothner AD: Valproic acid: a review of 23 fatal cases. Ann Neurol 10:287, 1985

Strull WM, Lo B, Charles G: Do patients want to participate in medical decision making? JAMA 252:2990–2994, 1984

Thurston JH, Hauhart RE: Chronic valproate induces key enzymes of hepatic fatty acid oxidation and ketogenesis in infant mice. Pediatric Res 1987 (in press)

Vaccarino JM: Consent, informed consent and the consent form. N Engl J Med 298:455, 1978

Weiss G, Hechtman LT: Hyperactive Children Grown Up. New York, Guilford Press, 1986

Wiener JM (ed): Diagnosis and Psychopharmacology of Childhood and Adolescent Disorders. New York, John Wiley & Sons, 1985

Zafrani ES, Berthelot P: Sodium valproate in the induction of unusual hepatotoxicity. Hepatology 2:648–649, 1982

Zimmerman HJ, Ishak KG: Valproate-induced hepatic injury: analysis of 23 fatal cases. Hepatology 2:591–597, 1982